Ninety-Nine Lessons in Critical Thinking

Ninety-Nine Lessons in Critical Thinking

Robert P. Friedland, MD

Rudd Chair and Professor, Departments of Neurology and Anatomy and Neurobiology
University of Louisville School of Medicine
Louisville, KY, USA

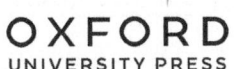

OXFORD
UNIVERSITY PRESS

Oxford University Press is a department of the University of Oxford.
It furthers the University's objective of excellence in research, scholarship,
and education by publishing worldwide. Oxford is a registered trade mark of
Oxford University Press in the UK and certain other countries.

Published in the United States of America by Oxford University Press
198 Madison Avenue, New York, NY 10016, United States of America.

© Oxford University Press 2025

All rights reserved. No part of this publication may be reproduced, stored in a retrieval system,
transmitted, used for text and data mining, or used for training artificial intelligence, in any form or
by any means, without the prior permission in writing of Oxford University Press, or as expressly
permitted by law, by license or under terms agreed with the appropriate reprographics rights
organization. Inquiries concerning reproduction outside the scope of the above should be sent
to the Rights Department, Oxford University Press, at the address above.

You must not circulate this work in any other form
and you must impose this same condition on any acquirer

CIP data is on file at the Library of Congress

ISBN 978-0-19-775621-8

This material is not intended to be, and should not be considered, a substitute for medical or other
professional advice. Treatment for the conditions described in this material is highly dependent on the
individual circumstances. And, while this material is designed to offer accurate information with respect
to the subject matter covered and to be current as of the time it was written, research and knowledge about
medical and health issues is constantly evolving and dose schedules for medications are being revised
continually, with new side effects recognized and accounted for regularly. Readers must therefore always
check the product information and clinical procedures with the most up-to-date published product
information and data sheets provided by the manufacturers and the most recent codes of conduct and
safety regulation. The publisher and the authors make no representations or warranties to readers, express
or implied, as to the accuracy or completeness of this material. Without limiting the foregoing, the
publisher and the authors make no representations or warranties as to the accuracy or efficacy of the drug
dosages mentioned in the material. The authors and the publisher do not accept, and expressly disclaim,
any responsibility for any liability, loss, or risk that may be claimed or incurred as a consequence of the use
and/ or application of any of the contents of this material.

DOI: 10.1093/med/9780197756218.001.0001

Printed by Integrated Books International, United States of America

The manufacturer's authorised representative in the EU for product safety is
Oxford University Press España S.A. of el Parque Empresarial San Fernando
de Henares, Avenida de Castilla, 2 - 28830 Madrid (www.oup.es/en)

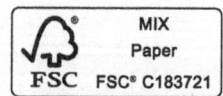

To Shivani, the most wondrous and insightful person I have ever known.

Ami tomake bhalobasi

Preconceived ideas are like searchlights which illume the path of the experimenter and serve her as a guide to interrogate nature. They become a danger only if she transports transforms them into fixed ideas—this is why I should like to see these profound words inscribed on the threshold of all the temples of science: the greatest derangement of the mind is to believe in something because one wishes it to be so.

—Louis Pasteur (adapted)

Contents

Preface   xiii
Acknowledgments   xvii

SECTION I DOCTOR–PATIENT INTERACTIONS

1. The World Is Too Complex To Perceive Directly   3
2. The Key Factor Which Determines What We Perceive Is Our Attention and How It Is Focused   6
3. Which Is Older, Stories or Books?   9
4. Be Fierce, Nurture an Intense and Ferocious Aggressiveness in the Pursuit of Your Learning and the Benefit of Your Patients   11
5. "Listen to Your Patient, He Is Telling You the Diagnosis"   16
6. Be a Good Observer   19
7. Consider the Patient's Experience   21
8. Learn from Your Patients   24
9. Intellectualization Limits Your Compassion   26
10. Key Elements of the Patient Visit: The Interview and Deep Listening   29
11. Words Influence Thought   33
12. The Physical Exam   37
13. Touch Is Important   39
14. Be Prepared for the Unexpected   41

SECTION II DIAGNOSIS AND EVALUATION

15. The Fundamental Three-Step Approach to Diagnosis   45
16. A Mnemonic for Etiologies, VITAMINS ABCD   47
17. Investigations   49
18. Don't Be Afraid To Say You Don't Know   51

19. Information Toxicity — 54
20. Treat the Patient, Not the Test — 56
21. It's Good To Be Knowledgeable, but It Is Necessary to Also Be Attentive to the Patient — 58
22. Consider Toxic Exposures — 60
23. Family History Is an Important Part of the Interview — 62
24. Rare Presentations of Common Events Are More Common Than Common Presentations of Rare Events — 63
25. Symptoms and Signs Have Important Significance: The Absence of Symptoms and Signs Is Not Always as Important as Their Presence — 64
26. Salutogenesis: The Production and Maintenance of Health — 66

SECTION III MANAGEMENT

27. Get to Know the Patient and Show Interest (the Patient Is a Person) — 71
28. Learn from Clinical Experience (but Not Too Much) — 74
29. Use the Placebo Response to Your Patient's Benefit — 75
30. Tell the Truth Whenever Possible — 76
31. Cognitive Function Is Relevant for All Areas of Medicine — 78
32. You Are Primarily Responsible for Caring for the Patient, Not the Family — 79
33. Denial of Illness and Disability Can Be Shared by the Patient, the Family, and the Doctor — 80
34. Consider the Context of Care — 82
35. Challenges to the Ability to Provide Humane Healthcare — 86
36. Do Not Confuse Etiology with Pathophysiology — 90
37. Communicate with the Patient — 92
38. Be Attentive to Medications and Medication Errors — 94

SECTION IV CRITICAL THINKING

39. Think Deeply (Think Beyond the Obvious) — 99
40. How Often Do Rare Events Occur? — 104

41. Do Not Depend on Logic Alone	107
42. Although Intuition Cannot Replace Evidence, It Can Be Valuable	110
43. Should You Think Out of the Box?	112
44. All Models Are Wrong	114
45. Biomarkers Are Not the Disease Itself	116
46. Absence of Evidence Is Not Evidence of Absence	118
47. Being Wrong (at Times) Is OK	122
48. Much of What We Know Is Wrong (So Don't Believe Everything You Read)	124
49. Smart People Make Mistakes	126
50. Fishing Expeditions May Be Productive	129
51. Manifestations of Bias	131
52. Experimenter Bias	141
53. Bias of the Lost Actors	143
54. Being Smart Is Not Enough	144
55. Don't Be Afraid of Your Imagination	146
56. Do Not Assume That Your Ideas Are Not Novel and Important Just Because They Appear To Be Obvious	149
57. Consider the Evolutionary Aspects of Disease	151

SECTION V PERSONAL AND CAREER DEVELOPMENT

58. Live in "Day-Tight Compartments"	157
59. Learn How to Learn and Enhance Your Learning Capacity	159
60. Find Out Where You Find Meaning	163
61. Search for Your Passion and Follow It (Gnaw Your Own Bone)	165
62. Learn to Critically Read the Literature	168
63. We Are All Neurologists	170
64. Neurology and Cardiology (Etc.) Don't Exist	172
65. Do Not Respect Boundaries, Be a Trespasser	174

66. Be Grateful	176
67. Look Beyond the Easiest Options and Pursue the Best Resources Possible	178
68. Focus, but Not Too Much	180
69. Be Persistent and Tenacious	182
70. Do Not Be Intimidated by Accomplished Persons in Medicine and Science	185
71. Accept the Help of Others	187
72. Pay Attention to Your Own Health and Learn How To Deal with Stress	190
73. Learn from the History of Medicine and Science	193
74. Recognize Your Intellectual Ancestors	196
75. You Are an Educator—That's One of Your Most Important Responsibilities	198
76. Learn To Be a Salesperson	200
77. Learn How To Learn from Bad Example	202
78. Remember Pierre Curie, Carl Wernicke, and Others	203

SECTION VI DISCOVERY

79. What Is Science?	207
80. No Single Theory Ever Agrees with All the Facts	211
81. There Is Only One Kind of Science, and That Is the Study of Everything with All Possible Methods	214
82. It's Good To Be First, but It Is Not Necessary	216
83. You Don't Need To Be Brilliant To Be a Researcher	219
84. Appreciate a Diversity of Approaches	221
85. Why Think When You Can Experiment?	224
86. Judge Every Project by Asking "What Difference Will It Make To Know the Answer?"	228
87. What Is Important in Research	230
88. Do Not Be Obsessed with Technology and Methods	232

89. Pay Attention to Study Design, Data Analysis, and Statistics	235
90. Be Aware of (*Beware of*) Statistics and Data Torturing	238
91. Pay Attention to the Assumptions of Diagnostic Testing and Research Evaluations	240
92. It Is Possible To Be Productive from a Distance	243
93. You Can Make Contributions as a Clinician Without a Laboratory	245

SECTION VII ETHICS

94. Never Whisper in the Presence of Wrong	249
95. You Are Responsible for Your Actions; You Cannot Let Others Take Responsibility for You	252
96. The Need To Believe in the Guilty Victim	255
97. Compassion Is Part of Our Fundamental Nature	257
98. The Myth of Progress	259
99. Don't Be Ageist	261
Epilogue	265
Quotations on the Nature of the Scientific Endeavor	269
About the Author	271
Index	273

Preface

There are some things I would like you to know. The practice of medicine and scientific investigation involve a massive amount of information, now more than ever. There is danger that the needs of the patient will be buried by this knowledge. Also, in all scientific endeavors, there are more data available than ever before. There is a risk that these data will cloud your reasoning and decision-making.

The main goal of this book is to help you to be aware of your own thinking and reasoning processes so that you can best understand the story of the patient and the story of your investigative work. I would like you to pay attention to your own cognition—how you learn, how you remember, how you observe, how you make decisions, and how you use your powers of attention. You need to pay attention to your own thinking as well as to the patient and to the scientific problem at hand. Another principal goal of this book is to help young doctors and researchers recognize the humanity of both the patient and themselves.

This book is aimed at both doctors and scientists. When I refer to doctors, I include physicians, scientists, dentists, nurse practitioners, nurses, psychologists, and other healthcare providers. The work is also targeted at scientists of all kinds, including those involved in medicine as well as those in other disciplines. I am also hopeful that laypersons will be interested in learning about critical thinking.

Critical thinking involves paying attention to your questioning and to your thinking. Many of our thoughts are produced while our mind is on autopilot. Physicist Georg Lichtenberg (1742–1799) said "we think early in life but we do not know we are thinking, any more than we know we are growing or digesting; Many ordinary people never do discover it." This is certainly true about most of us.

Critical thinking assists in comprehensively evaluating evidence for both medical and other scientific matters. It helps put things in perspective so you can evaluate what is important and what is not. Also, critical thinking involves respect for all forms of thinking: logical, rational, and intuitive. It's important to carefully consider how the questions are phrased and what implications may be implied. What do the words in the question really mean? How is our understandings of the questions influenced by the way the words are chosen and how the argument is framed? And how are our biases involved in forming our questions and analyzing situations and data?

Do we welcome our questioning and the questioning of others, or are we content in believing what we've been taught and what we've always believed? "To know how to wonder and question is the first step of the mind toward discovery," according to Louis Pasteur.

Critical thinking does not need to be attacking or finding fault. It can be complementary and assist in the creation of good arguments. Finding fault is easy; building consensus and new ideas is harder. And, of course, being critical applies to your own ideas as well as those of others.

There are no magical formulas for applying critical thinking. It involves the consideration of available evidence and forming judgments based on rational analysis. And it is essential for problem-solving.

I believe that this book will assist you in becoming a better doctor and scientist through focus on your capacity for attention, compassion, reasoning, judgment, and observation. I'd like to assist you in developing your appreciation of the many factors which influence reasoning. It is critical to be aware of our own thought processes and to understand how language and preconceived ideas can influence observation, experimentation, and data analysis. This book will help you advance through consideration of how the mind processes information and how our perceptual processes are related to our thoughts and ideas.

For much of the time, our actions and reactions develop automatically, without much thought. This is true in our private lives as well as in our professional lives as doctors and scientists. We learn what to do in certain situations, and, when these situations appear, we do what we have always done. The inconvenient truth is that thinking can be difficult. Many people don't like to do it, and it is generally easier to avoid thinking and instead rely upon "autopilot." According to linguist Noam Chomsky, "people not only don't know what's happening to them, they don't even know that they don't know."

This book is comprised of lessons that I have learned over four and a half decades of teaching, clinical care, and research. My experience is that teaching is usually devoted to facts that must be learned for exams. This book is focused on the important concepts that a young doctor or scientist must learn and that they will not learn from a textbook or from a classroom. I wish to help people to become observant, compassionate, thoughtful, and caring doctors and scientists. **It is necessary that you unlearn the focus on "facts" and learn to think about your thinking and consider how you know what you know.**

This book presents ideas about thought and judgment which are supported by examples from my own life as well as from history and literature. The stories are chosen because of the principles they demonstrate. I believe that the stories offered are informative as well as enjoyable. Frequently, more than one story is presented to demonstrate a particular point in order to better express the principle involved.

References to the history of science and history of medicine are frequently used throughout the book. We need to understand that people are largely the same today as they were in the past few hundred years. Human evolution has expanded the cognitive capacity of the brain, largely through the growth of the frontal lobes, over the past few 100,000 years. However, there has been only limited evolutionary changes in the brain in the past few hundred years of human history. Our ancestors who thought that the Sun revolved around the Earth did not suffer from some deficit of brain structure which prevented them from realizing the true relationship of the Sun and the

Earth. Humans today are certainly capable of such widespread misconceptions. The fact that much of what we know is wrong is powerfully illustrated by history.

The study of the history of medicine and science shows us how important it is to be aware of our biases, preconceived ideas, and errors of reasoning. We also need to be aware of the powerful role of language in framing our reasoning. History illustrates the importance of thinking for ourselves and appreciating the enormous power of our imagination.

This book is not a textbook, and it is not an academic treatise on critical thinking. If you are interested in learning the names of the 12 cranial nerves, how to read an electrocardiogram, or the appropriate dose of penicillin for a 11-year-old with a strep throat, there are many excellent resources available. This book will not help you address these aspects of your education. Furthermore, this book will not tell you how to repair a fractured hip, but it will suggest that you consider what could be the reasons why the hip was fractured and also help you attend to the person with the fracture, not just the broken bone. This book will not tell you what the best antibiotic is for pneumococcal pneumonia, but it will discuss how attention to compliance (how well patients follow instructions concerning drugs) is often a matter of life and death. This book will not tell you how to do a Western blot or how to do a polymerase chain reaction assay, but it will help you understand the significance of the molecular data. This book will not provide you with the direct clinical experiences you need but will help you to pay attention to the patient as a person so that you can use the power of stories as a potent enhancer of learning.

The electronic health record and artificial intelligence are having profound influences on patient care. The ability to retain focus on the patient must be maintained, even in the modern clinical environment with its extensive availability of information. Although modern computer resources are enormously valuable, they can obscure the reality of the patient's needs and experience. We must learn to use these resources to help us better provide person-centered care. Note that I have referred to the need to provide the best "person-centered care." I'm not referring to the need for "patient-centered care" because patients are persons who have already been identified as needing medical help. It is much more effective for healthcare to focus on persons through the provision of preventive measures.

My patients have taught me most of what I know. I share their stories, which are the most powerful tools of learning. I hope that you find these stories valuable, and I trust that this book will enhance your mission of becoming an outstanding physician and scientist.

I illustrate important points in the book with quotations. The lives of historically important physicians and scientists that are mentioned will be briefly summarized in headings called "A Person to Know." Stories of cases may contain adjustments that are needed to maintain confidentiality. References are provided to complement the text and to direct you to valuable sources of further information.

The opinions expressed in the book are my own. Undoubtedly you will come upon ideas that I propose with which you disagree. Some of my positions are certainly contrary to established beliefs in the scientific community. I eagerly propose that you form your own opinions.

The lessons presented in the book are not ordered with regard to importance, although the book is designed to be read in the order in which the lessons are provided. The book can also be read without regard to this order. I am is grateful for the model provided by Edward O. Wilson of Harvard University, author of *Letters to Young Scientists*.[1]

> Education is not the filling of a vessel, rather it is the lighting of the fire.
> —Attributed to Plutarch, Greek philosopher

> A good example has twice the value as good advice.
> —Albert Schweitzer (1875–1965)

Reference

1. Wilson EO. *Letters to Young Scientists*. W.W. Norton; 2013.

Acknowledgments

The author is grateful for the continual support and affection of his wife Shivani Nandi who has assisted in the publication of this work in countless ways.

The author is very appreciative of the strong foundation of independent thought which he received from his mentors Morris B. Bender and Edwin A. Weinstein at the Mount Sinai School of Medicine in New York.

The author is also grateful for the support of the University of Louisville, the Michael J. Fox Foundation, the family of Edward A. Ford III, the Mason and Mary Rudd family, the Jewish Heritage Fund for Excellence, and the Kentucky Science and Engineering Foundation.

The author is especially appreciative of important discussions with Douglas Rothenberg, Arthur Hoffmann, and Peter Lauf. He is also thankful for comments about an earlier version of the work from Megan Coghlan, Martin Brown, Ruma Rahachowdhury, Sudeep Basu, Karen and Mark Robinson, Qi Dai, and Demetra Antimisiaris.

SECTION I
DOCTOR–PATIENT INTERACTIONS

Lesson 1
The World Is Too Complex To Perceive Directly

Our sensory systems, including visual, somatosensory (touch, pain, temperature), auditory, gustatory, olfactory, and vestibular (balance) functions, did not evolve to allow us to perceive the world the way it really is. This task would be much too difficult for the processing capacity of any nervous system. Our senses are highly developed and skillful, but they do not show the world to us in its completeness. We cannot assess the presence of air in a baby's stomach the way a dolphin's mother can. We cannot find our way around in the dark, as can a bat. Humans are able to perceive only a narrow segment of the electromagnetic spectrum (visible light). Our ability to experience our environment is vastly different from that of a dolphin or a bat.*

Our sensory abilities evolved to enhance our survival and augment the survival of our children. Human evolution is based on the preferred dissemination of genes which help survival. Sensory capacities which help us to see the electric fields of flowers would not have been helpful for the survival of our ancestors (such a skill is important for insects, however). We can see only a small part of the solar spectrum, and our ears can perceive only a small part of the sounds available (just ask a bat, a whale or a dolphin). On the other hand, noticing the slight movement of a predator is quite valuable. Humans, as well as most other vertebrates, have a visual system with great sensitivity to movement.[2] Our perceptions are not based on comprehensive analysis of all the features of all possible stimuli. Rather, we are constantly making estimates (guesses) about what is happening. These concepts are described in the book *The Case Against Reality: How Evolution Hid the Truth from Our Eyes* by cognitive scientist Donald Hoffman.[3]

Homo sapiens is a relatively new species on Earth, with a history dating back only about 100,000 years. In comparison, our nearest relative, the chimpanzee, has been around about 6–7 million years (60 times longer than us). For most of this past our primate ancestors lived in a very different environment than the one we live in today. Our genes were selected in that environment because they helped us to survive at that time. Therefore, we must realize that we have not had the opportunity to develop new genes to assist us specifically in the modern world with cell phones, computers, and enormous demands on our processing capacity.

---

* The implications of the unique nature of our experience of the world for our understanding of consciousness is discussed in an important 1974 paper, "What is it like to be a bat" by philosopher Thomas Nagel.[1]

Imagine an ancient ancestor of ours going out in search of water. (It is only in the twentieth century that many people on Earth had good access to water.) Our water-seeking relative walks through her forest habitat and hears the sound of flowing water. As she approaches the creek, she must be aware that predators also need to drink. Our ancestor should not process the varying shades of green of all the leaves available in her sight. She also should not mentally measure the relative height of all the trees and the relative size of all the flowers. Rather, she needs to be attentive to things that are moving and for sounds that may indicate the presence of another being.

Similarly, when we drive a car in the city we cannot observe and mentally catalog the clothing of all the pedestrians, what kind of shoes are they wearing, and the font used in the signs in the stores. How many pedestrians have sandals and how many sneakers? Are they wearing socks? We must focus on the road, other cars, pedestrians, and traffic signals. Our expectations provide us with a powerful filter that enhances our perception of environmental stimuli that we need to notice.

This means that we do not see the world the way it really is: we see it through our expectations of what may be happening. The brain analyzes what it observes and makes conclusions based on past experience. Our conclusions about what is or is not happening is not based on the analysis of everything in our perceptual experience. This is well expressed by the great Harvard psychologist William James, who said, **"The art of being wise is knowing what to overlook."**

Being a good observer is a necessary skill for healthcare workers. A good observer is not one who observes everything and processes all available information. Rather, being a good observer means having knowledge of the reality that we cannot process everything, that we all have a powerful filter, and that there will be things that we ignore. Awareness of this process is critical for medicine and science.

Attention is a vital component of awareness. To paraphrase the English writer Aldous Huxley, "Experience is not what happens to us, experience is what we do with what happens to us." William James (here he is again) pointed out that a pack of dogs let loose for a year in the British Museum in London would not learn anything about art. The canines would experience the art but would not pay attention to it. Our ability to make clinical and scientific observations is based on our use of this power of attention.

Rather than perceive the world the way it really is, we perceive it according to what we expect. Awareness, attention, expectations, and overlooking all provide an opportunity for bias to influence perceptions. A critical point of this book is that we cannot solve these matters directly. We cannot begin to see the world exactly the way it is because that's not possible. We also cannot perceive the world without ignoring parts of it—that's just not possible. We cannot pay attention to everything in our world—that is also not attainable. Furthermore, we cannot experience the world without any bias whatsoever—that's not possible. What we need is awareness that attention, expectations, and bias influence our experience of the world. This awareness is critical.

As Nobel Prize–winning immunologist Gerald Edelman, with coauthor Giulio Tononi, has said "If our view of memory is correct, in higher organisms every act of perception is, to some degree, an act of creation, and every act of memory is, to some degree, an act of imagination."[4]

You can observe a lot by watching.

—Yogi Berra, American baseball player[5]

The brain evolved into its present form over a period of about two million years, from the time of *Homo habilis* to the late stone age of *Homo sapiens,* during which people existed in hunter-gatherer bands in intimate contact with the natural environment. Snakes mattered. The smell of water, the hum of a bee, the directional adaptive: the glimpse of one small animal hidden in the grass could make the difference between eating and going hungry in the evening. And a sweet sense of horror, the shivery fascination with monsters and creeping forms that so delights us today even in the sterile hearts of the cities, could see you through to the next morning. Organisms are the natural stuff of metaphor and ritual. Although the evidence is far from all in, the brain appears to have kept its old capacities, its channeled quickness. We stay alert and alive in the vanished forests of the world.

—Edward O. Wilson[2]

Edward O. Wilson (1929-2021): A Person to Know

American evolutionary biologist and entomologist. He was the founder of the field of sociobiology and authored numerous books on the influence of evolution on culture and social behavior. Two of his books won Pulitzer Prizes. He wrote numerous books on insects, biodiversity, and conservation. His book *Biophilia* describes the evolutionary origin of the love people have for natural things. He was also the author of *Consilience: The Unity of Knowledge.*[†]

References

1. Nagel T. What is it like to be a bat? *Philosoph Rev.* 1974;83(4):435–50.
2. Wilson EO. *Biophilia.* Harvard University Press; 2003.
3. Hoffman D. *The Case Against Reality: How Evolution Hid the Truth from Our Eyes.* Norton; 2019.
4. Edelman GM, Tononi G. *A Universe of Consciousness: How Matter Becomes Imagination.* Basic Books; 2001.
5. Berra Y. *You Can Observe a Lot by Watching.* Turner Publishing; 2009.

[†] "Consilience" refers to the harmony of knowledge obtained from various modes of exploration. Some of Wilson's opinions have been criticized for the support of pseudoscience.

Lesson 2
The Key Factor Which Determines What We Perceive Is Our Attention and How It Is Focused

[H]ow false (is) a notion of experience that ... would make it tantamount to the mere presence to the senses of an outward order. Millions of items of the outward order are present to my senses which never properly enter into my experience. Why? Because they have no interest for me. *My experience is what I agree to attend to.* Only those items which I notice shape my mind—without selective interest, experience is an utter chaos. Interest alone gives accent and emphasis, light and shade, background and foreground-intelligible perspective, in a word. It varies in every creature, but without it, the consciousness of every creature would be a gray chaotic indiscriminativeness, impossible for us even to conceive.

—William James (emphasis added)[1]

As discussed in the first lesson, the world is much too complicated for any organism to perceive everything that is available to its nervous system. Rather than sense the world as it really is, we have evolved a system of complex expectations. Our nervous system analyzes the world and finds the best explanations for what it notices. If you are walking in a forest in Connecticut and an animal is seen moving up a tree, a squirrel will be expected, not an orangutang. If I say the sentence "John went to the library and came home with a book," your brain will have accurately predicted that the last word in the sentence was going to be "book" based on the first words in the sentence. This unconscious linguistic process takes place very quickly and is based on experience. That is, it's possible that the sentence could have been "John went to the library and came home with a wildebeest," but this outcome is highly unlikely. We are only able to read at all because our nervous system can anticipate successfully. If we had to read each word in a book our reading abilities would be painful and torpid.

Our dependence on expectations is illustrated by this paragraph:

Aoccdrnig to a rscheearch at Cmabrigde Uinervtisy, it deosn't mttaer in waht oredr the ltteers in a wrod are, the olny iprmoetnt tihng is taht the frist and lsat ltteer be at the rghit pclae. The rset can be a toatl mses and you can sitll raed it wouthit porbelm. Tihs is bcuseae the huamn mnid deos not raed ervey lteter by istlef, but the wrod as a wlohe.[2]

Even though most words are misspelled we can understand the paragraph because of our expectations. This is because the human mind does not read every letter by itself, but the word in the context of the sentence.

The dependence of perception on expectations is also illustrated by the monkey business illusion, in which a gorilla is not noticed because of attention directed elsewhere.[3]

What you experience depends on the expectations that are set up in the situation and its context. If you are on call at night and a new admission comes in and you are asked to see the patient with the instructions from your senior resident "go see the new stroke in room 37B," you should be aware that your improperly set expectation that the patient has a stroke may lead you to have preconceived ideas which influence your interactions with the patient. (It is also improper to refer to a person by the name of their disease. This inhumane practice was common in medical education 50 years ago.)

The role of experience in perception is illustrated by a story from Colin Turnbull's anthropological classic *The Forest People*.[4] He took Kenge, a young Mbuti pygmy who grew up in the jungle of central Africa, to the eastern African savanna. The man had limited experience of seeing things which were a great distance away, and he had not learned that large things that are far away appear to be small. When he saw a buffalo that was at a distance, he tried to catch it with his hand because he thought it was a fly.*

We are not perceiving everything that we experience but rather constantly estimating probabilities and preparing expectations. These estimations are determined by our past experience and by our filters. It's not possible or desirable to turn off these cognitive mechanisms. What is necessary is to be aware of them.

Our ability to interact with patients depends on our ability to focus our attention on the patient. I had an 82-year-old female patient who was concerned about her memory. I performed a comprehensive evaluation and told her that her minor memory problems were not surprising considering her age and were not indicative of Alzheimer's disease. Because of lumbar disc disease she had unstable gait and used a tripod cane. I noticed that she was wearing shoes with 2-inch heels. (Stability is enhanced by contact with the ground.) I said to her "I'm very sorry but I must recommend that at your age and with your instability you should not wear high-heeled shoes." She said to me "But Dr. Friedland, I was coming to see you!" My observation of her inappropriate footwear may have saved her a fall and a hip fracture as well as associated risk of pneumonia and death.

The setting of the patient interaction needs to be controlled to allow for attention to the patient. On one occasion I visited a physician as a patient to discuss operative options for my care. He spent all the time in the consultation focused on his computer, which allowed me an excellent view only of his left ear. I decided that I could not allow

---

* The man was also shown a person water skiing in a lake and asked, "Why is the boat attempting to escape from the man?"

a surgeon to operate on me if he couldn't maintain eye contact. It is necessary for the computer to be placed so that it can be viewed at the same time as the patient.

> We don't see things as they are. We see things as we are.
> —Attributed to Anais Nin, French American author

> Experience is not what happens to a woman; it is what a woman does with what happens to her.
> —Aldous Huxley (1894–1953, English author
> (adapted from *Texts and Pretexts*)[5]

William James (1842–1910): A Person to Know

William James was an American psychologist and philosopher who was the first to offer a course in psychology. He was a physician who taught anatomy at Harvard University but never practiced medicine. James helped establish the philosophical schools of pragmatism and empiricism. He was the brother of the prominent novelist Henry James and the writer Alice James. His highly influential *Principles of Psychology* (1890) was the most important text in the discipline for many decades. James's 1902 book, *The Varieties of Religious Experience: A Study of Human Nature*, is one of the earliest explorations of individual spiritual experiences as well as mysticism across diverse cultural traditions.

References

1. James W. *The Principles of Psychology*. Henry Holt; 1890.
2. MRC Cognition and Brain Sciences Unit. January 2008. http://www.mrc-cbu.cam.ac.uk/~mattd/Cmabrigde/. Accessed Nov 2, 2023.
3. EPEC. *Education for Physicians Participants Handbook, Module 2, Communicating Bad News*. Robert Wood Johnson Foundation; 1991.
4. Turnbull C. *The Forest People*. Touchstone; 1987.
5. Huxley A. *Texts and Pretexts*. Chatto & Windus; 1932.

Lesson 3
Which Is Older, Stories or Books?

This incredibly easy question is meant to illustrate a critical point. Our brains developed through evolution with a powerful capacity for learning through stories. For almost all of human history information was exchanged through stories, not books. It is only in the twentieth century that many people in the world became able to read. And, of course, books are only a few hundred years old. For the vast majority of the 100,000 years of human history our ancestors depended on stories to learn about their world. This information transmitted with stories contained vital knowledge which was critical for survival.

Imagine a family living 50,000 years ago who had a child who, because of a unique combination of genes, had no interest in stories. As a result, she didn't pay attention when information was passed down about what the clan did during periods of drought. When she grew up, she had a survival disadvantage when a drought came, and she would be less likely to pass on her genetically influenced disinterest in stories than a sibling with an intense interest in the clan's stories.

This evolutionary phenomenon is no doubt responsible for the enormous variety of books, movies, and other media available to us today. The appetite for stories is quite remarkable: it is estimated that British mystery writer Agatha Christie has sold more than 2 billion books. **The brain is made for the processing of stories. Our appreciation of this truth can help to enhance our learning and improve the quality of our patient care.**

What does this have to do with the practice of medicine? We must respect the patient's stories, and we must turn our learning into stories whenever possible. Appreciating the power of stores will enhance our ability to think critically and ask good questions. If we read in a book that the innervation of muscles of the lower face by the seventh cranial nerve is mostly crossed and the innervation of the upper face is both crossed and uncrossed, we may very well remember these facts. If we see this demonstrated in a patient, this becomes a part of your own story of the patient and it becomes a more salient (significant) memory. It is also valuable to consider this from a perceptual point of view. If you read a fact in a book, the input is purely visual. If you see a patient, your experience has visual, auditory, and tactile components. Clearly the brain is better at making memories that involve more than one perceptual modality. Additionally, every patient represents a story. This is not true of every fact read in the book. Every patient has a story about their presentation to our care, and, from the point of view of the physician, every patient is a story.

Similarly, we must allow the patient to experience the medical encounter as a story based on human terms. We must respect their story and help them appreciate the story that we give them about their condition. This attention and respect will improve their ability to do what we would like them to do. It is not enough to tell the patient what you want them to do and then dismiss them with, "You can go now." Rather, you must explain what you want them to do, why they should do it, what may happen if they do it, what might happen if they don't do it, and how these instructions fit into the fabric of their lives. You must explain how your instructions aligns with the context of their care (e.g., it won't help for you to tell the patient what treatment is needed if they lack the resources to obtain it; see Lesson 34).[1]

For example, I often recommend that patients lower their consumption of sugar. I do not restrict my advice to the production of a list (such as don't do A, B, C, D, E, F, and G). Rather, I tell them that excess sugar consumption enhances inflammation in the body through actions on bacteria in the intestine which have damaging influences throughout the body, including the brain. Also, I explain that excess sugar consumption is a risk factor for diabetes, obesity, stroke, and heart disease. I explain how sugar consumption can be lowered (what dietary choices they should make), and I give them concrete examples (e.g., do not put sugar on your cereal in the morning, but rather raisins, which have natural sweetness and also beneficial fiber). I may also explain how successful management of their metabolic problems may enhance their fitness, longevity, and ability to do things that they find meaningful (such as playing golf or attending their granddaughter's high school graduation).

> Every time I see a new patient, I read a new book.
> —**Toshikazu Yoshikawa (President of the Louis Pasteur Center for Medical Research. Kyoto, Japan; personal communication)**

Reference

1. Weiner SJ, Schwartz A, *Listening for What Matters: Avoiding Contextual Errors in Health Care*. Oxford University Press; 2016.

Lesson 4
Be Fierce, Nurture an Intense and Ferocious Aggressiveness in the Pursuit of Your Learning and the Benefit of Your Patients

The word "fierce" comes from the Latin *ferus* or "untamed." It is necessary to be fierce in the pursuit of your own learning. And also to be fierce in working for the benefit of the patients. As we have seen in the first two lessons, we do not learn from experience; we learn from the focusing of our attention. If you go to a lecture, sit in the back of the room as far away from the lecturer as possible, and listen as you tend to your email, you may learn something. If you choose to sit in the front and follow the facial expressions of the lecturer and ask questions to enhance your understanding, you will learn more. If you sit at home studying, read a 30-page chapter in a textbook, and come upon the anatomical localization of pain commonly seen in appendicitis you may remember it well. If you see it demonstrated by a patient contorted in pain in the emergency room, you will never forget it.

The ability to demonstrate ferocity as a student, either in medical school, graduate school, or elsewhere, is often actively inhibited by institutions. Programs may leave little time for questions. Professors often do not wish to have their teaching questioned or their opinions challenged. Faculty productivity may be impaired when students ask questions. Moreover, the role of the student may be directly forced into passivity by labeling the activity as "shadowing." As discussed in Lesson 11, the choice of words influence how we think (framing). There is nothing more passive than a shadow!

> Most of the time, if you speak up, at least 30% of the people in the room will have the same question and weren't brave enough to ask it. There are no stupid questions.
> —Nicola Fox, Associate Administrator for NASA's Science Mission Directorate, NASA Head of Science[1]

If you see a clinical finding illustrated by a patient, write it down in a little book which you keep in your pocket at all times, and read about the event that evening, the power of your memory will be enhanced enormously. Subjects can come up on rounds and at other times which are not effectively explained because of time pressures. If you write notes to yourself and read about them later, you will find your memory significantly enhanced. The great Johns Hopkins physician William Osler recommended the presence of these little books in doctor's pockets in his 1921 essay on the student life.[2]

If you are on a rotation in the emergency room and see a sick patient who is eventually admitted to the surgery service, you may not have the opportunity to see that patient again. However, if you can make time the next day to see what happened to that patient, you may learn that the diagnosis was wrong and that the plan for the patient had changed. This kind of experience is vital for your learning.

Young doctors are busy obtaining their clinical experience. The quality of these experiences is vital because it influences lifelong learning. **Activities in your early years form enduring patterns of learning and critical thinking that will influence the quality of care you provide throughout your career.** Our memories of the first time we did something are stronger than memories of other times. When your experience in a situation is limited, your processing of the experience is enhanced, and your memory (the story) is likely to be strong.

I suggest that you demonstrate ferocity in the pursuit of your learning.

Continuing with the theme of ferocity: you need to become familiar with the tools that are available to help you. This means that you cannot afford to be completely dependent on radiologists and laboratory professionals. If you are working in obstetrics and gynecology, you need to know how to interpret uterine ultrasound studies. If you are a cardiologist, you need to be able to analyze an echocardiogram. If you are a neurologist or neurosurgeon, you need to be able to evaluate an MRI scan of the brain. This does not mean that you will replace the radiologists, but you need to be able to form an opinion of your own. Your competence in interpreting these procedures will only come from experience. You may be surprised what you discover: One study found that when shown a chest X-ray of a patient missing a clavicle, 60% of radiologists failed to identify the missing bone.

It is equally important that you be fierce in the pursuit of your patient's benefit. You are their advocate. You are responsible for providing them with the best care possible. If you are not sure how to proceed with their care, you can refer them to other physicians. If you have uncertainty about a lab test, call the director of the laboratory. If you have question about a drug, call the pharmacist or call the drug company to have your question addressed. If you read a scientific paper and have a question, consider emailing the corresponding author of the paper to address your matters of concern.

Many years ago, I attended a dinner at a friend's house. He was upset that his brother had not arrived for dinner. (This was a time before cell phones.) The missing brother did not answer his home phone and did not come at all that evening. The next morning my friend called the police and found that his brother had had a car accident and a stroke and had been admitted to a local hospital. Because he was alone and did not have any information on him indicating who should be contacted, the brother had not been notified by the police or the hospital. Later that day my friend's brother died. It occurred to me that my friend's last name was unusual and if the doctor taking care of his brother had checked with the phone company, he would have found his family member's phone number, but he had not done so. This is an example of how ferocity in support of the patient's benefit could be helpful.

I was on call one night in an emergency room in Chinatown, in New York City. It was unusually quiet, and I wandered around wondering who would come in the door next when I noticed skull X-rays on the view box, I looked at the films and noted that they showed a skull fracture through the temporal bone. This is a particularly dangerous fracture because of the risk of epidural hematoma, which is a potentially deadly form of intracranial hemorrhage. I found that the patient had come in alone with a head injury a few hours before I arrived and had seen another doctor who did not notice the skull fracture and sent him home. (The fracture was obvious. When I showed the skull X-ray to my mother she identified the fracture right away. And she was not a radiologist.) I was concerned for the risk of bleeding, and I called the phone number listed for the patient and found that the number was not valid. I called the police and ask them to go to his address to explain to the patient that a mistake had been made and that he should come to the hospital urgently. They did so and found that there was no such address. The patient had not wanted us to know who he was, perhaps because of an altercation with police. In any event, he could not be located. The decision to call the police to look for him is an indication of a fierce attempt to provide care.

Similarly, if you see a patient who comes in being found down on the street without any informants, you need to work to find family members or friends who can tell you about the patient. On occasion I have asked family members to bring me the contents of the patient's medicine cabinet if the patient is not able to report what they are taking and there is possibility of drug interactions.

Raymond Adams and Maurice Victor of Harvard University contributed important early work on the neurological effects of alcohol abuse. Some patients were believed to be alcoholic even though they denied it, and Adams and Victor wanted to verify their level of alcohol intake for their research. One patient who asserted that he did not drink was offered a shot of whiskey at the bedside and downed it without hesitation. In another case, a neurologist went to a bar near the house of a patient who denied drinking with the patient's photograph and asked the bartender if he knew this fellow. The bartender said, "Of course, where has he been?" This is a good example of ferocity in patient care.

As examples of ferocity, I could have presented the important work of neurologist William Langston in discovering the molecular mechanism of a toxic form of Parkinson's disease (Lesson 46)[4] and also the Nobel Prize winning work of Barry Marshall and Robin Warren, who discovered the role of *Heliobacteria pylori* in peptic ulcer disease (Lesson 48).[5] But I have purposefully picked examples of "ferocity" in healthcare that are relatively simple to show that a high level of devotion to the patient does not require superhuman abilities. What is needed is a serious and tenacious commitment to the patient.[3]

Ferocity in the pursuit of scientific objectives is also necessary. There are countless examples that could be presented. Stanley Prusiner won the 1996 Nobel Prize in Physiology or Medicine "for his discovery of prions—a new biological principle of infection" (Lesson 82).[6] (Prions are abnormal transmissible disease agents that can induce pathogenic misfolding of host proteins). A key step in his discovery was his ability to sequence the prion protein in hamsters. His success was in part because he used many more animals than other researchers.

Daniel Carleton Gajdusek demonstrated the transmissibility of kuru, a degenerative disease of the brain, now shown to be caused by prions, which was transmitted by cannibalism in the eastern highlands of New Guinea. This work was accomplished through decades of living in the remote environment where the disease occurred. He learned the languages of the local tribes and obtained their collaboration through his tenacious efforts. He received the 1996 Nobel Prize in Physiology or Medicine for his work (Lesson 92).[7]

If you find the concept of ferocity inappropriate, consider the recommendation of Rudolph Virchow to "have icy enthusiasm." Harvard surgeon Atul Gawande agreed with the concept of ferocity. In his book *Better: A Surgeon's Notes on Performance*, he said "we want doctors who fight."[8] I considered using the word "tenacious" instead of "fierce," but I like the concept of aggressive and not only passive actions. Whatever terms we use it is critical that we are active and forceful in pursuing our learning and in helping patients under our care.

> The seemingly easiest and most sensible rule for a doctor to follow is: Always Fight. Always look for what more you could do.
> Atul Gawande, American surgeon and writer[8]

Sir William Osler (1849–1919): A Person to Know

Osler was a Canadian physician and one of the founding professors of the Johns Hopkins Hospital. He initiated the use of bedside clinical training and was a brilliant diagnostician and critical thinker. He was also active in originating residency training and introduced the clinicopathological method of teaching. His *Principles and Practice of Medicine*, first published in 1892, was the most prominent medicine textbook for more than 50 years and was translated into many languages.[9] Critically, he recognized both the biological and the human aspects of healthcare.[2,9]

Rudolph Virchow (1821–1902): A Person to Know

Virchow was a German physician and biologist. His work describing cellular pathology, published in 1851, showed that the cell is the fundamental unit of life. He demonstrated that each cell comes from another cell through cell division, and both disease and health originate through the cell. He is considered the founder of modern pathology as well as social medicine. Although his idea of the central importance of cellular pathology is correct, he did not accept Pasteur's germ theory. (It is reported that he did not like bacteriology.[10]) He was also an active anthropologist and politician and served in the German Reichstag (Parliament).

References

1. Geddes L. NASA's new Science chief Nicola Fox: "I grew up starstruck by space." *The Guardian*. 2013 Mar 17. https://www.theguardian.com/science/2023/mar/17/women-should-never-be-afraid-to-ask-questions-nasas-new-science-chief.
2. Osler W. A way of life and address to Yale students. 1913/2010. ReadaClassic.com.
3. Groopman J. *How Doctors Think*. Mariner Books; 2008, 179.
4. Langston JW, Palfreman J. *The Case of the Frozen Addicts* (2nd ed.). Pantheon Books; 2014.
5. Nobel Prize Organization. Barry Marshall Nobel Lecture. 2005. https://www.nobelprize.org/prizes/medicine/2005/marshall/lecture/
6. Prusiner SB. Novel proteinaceous infectious particles cause scrapie. *Science*. 1982 Apr 9;216(4542):136–44. doi:10.1126/science.6801762. PMID: 6801762.
7. Gajdusek DC, Gibbs CJ, Alpers M. Experimental transmission of a Kuru-like syndrome to chimpanzees. *Nature*. 1966 Feb 19;209(5025):794–6. doi:10.1038/209794a0. PMID: 5922150.
8. Gawande A. *Better: A Surgeon's Notes on Performance*. Henry Holt; 2007.
9. Osler W. *Principles and Practice of Medicine*. Forgotten Books Publishing; 2014, 71.
10. Hajdu SI. Rudolph Virchow, pathologist, armed revolutionist, politician, and anthropologist. *Ann Clin Lab Sci*. Spring 2005;35(2):203–5.

Lesson 5
"Listen to Your Patient, He Is Telling You the Diagnosis"

> Listen to your patient, he is telling you the diagnosis.
> —Attributed to William Osler

The best reason for listening to patients is that they may very well hold the key to the story of their illness. By knowing the nature of their symptoms—how they began, how they are changing with time, what makes them better, and what makes them worse, we may very well answer important questions about their diagnosis. This listening requires us to understand the patient's perspective on their experience of the symptoms. And this understanding requires us to get to know something about the patient as a person—not only the patient as a disease victim.

This listening is not passive, of course. It requires active and persistent questioning.

The need for this listening extends to all specialties in medicine. If you do not learn that your patient with a fever and rash has recently been to Africa, you may not consider performing the proper tests for certain infectious diseases. If you don't learn that the patient performs repetitive manual actions at work, you may not properly consider a diagnosis of peripheral nerve entrapment. Comprehensive listening can often remove the need for expensive and potentially hazardous diagnostic tests.

If the doctor doesn't listen it is unlikely that the patient will appreciate the sincerity of the doctor's concern. Many years ago, I injured my ankle and went to see a lower extremity specialist orthopedist. After spending an hour in the room waiting for him, he examined my ankle for 4 minutes and said that I needed an MRI as he exited the room. I angrily asked him where he was going because I had not yet told him the story of my ankle. I was upset that he did not appreciate the value of the story of my illness. The orthopedist could not think critically about my ankle if he didn't know how it was injured.

In a Veterans Administration hospital, I saw a 28-year-old man with loss of feeling on the fourth and fifth fingers of his left hand, hand weakness, and callus formation on the base of his thumb. Electromyography (EMG) and nerve conduction studies (electrical tests measuring nerve and muscle functions) showed damage to the ulnar nerve on the left. There was no reason to believe it was caused by trauma at work, and he did not have diabetes, which is a common cause of dysfunction of a peripheral nerve (neuropathy). A consulting neurosurgeon and I were perplexed about the cause of his condition until I asked him a pivotal question: What did he think was the cause? He said, "perhaps it was my addiction to playing a video game involving rolling a ball on the base of my thumb." He was doing it for hours every day. We published his case of "video-game palsy" in the *New England Journal of Medicine*.[1] I guess the joke should go, "How many physicians does it take to make a correct diagnosis?" Answer, "Only one who listens to the patient."

A 27-year-old man came to see me in clinic with pain on the right side of his neck radiating down over the right shoulder into his arm; the pain had been progressing over 1 month. There were no sensory deficit or motor findings (weakness). X-rays of his cervical spine was normal. When I asked him about his occupational and other activities, I could not find evidence of any concern. I was considering ordering an EMG study when I asked him if he had any idea what might be responsible for his pain. He said it might be a new yoga posture he had recently been practicing. I asked him to show me, and he climbed on the examining table and stood on his head with his neck bent with his feet in the air. I quickly said, "Don't do that." The spinal column in the neck is not capable of supporting the entire weight of the person when it is flexed or extended. His pain was relieved when he stopped adopting this posture, which is not a recommended part of a yoga practice.

There are many causes of dementia, which is a syndrome comprised of several cognitive difficulties including memory, judgment, verbal ability, route-finding, decision-making, and language. If you learn that a 72-year-old patient has had symptoms of dementia for 2 years which started slowly and are slowly progressive, a wide range of disorders may be responsible, such as Alzheimer's disease, the commonest cause of dementia worldwide. If you learned instead that the patients' cognitive problems started suddenly after they had a car accident with a head injury and loss of consciousness 2 years ago and since then has been getting better, you know that this is not Alzheimer's disease. Alzheimer's will not have a sudden onset and will not have 2 years of improvement.

If a 50-year-old person comes to the emergency room with a headache, you want to know if they have had headaches before and if this one is similar. Your management will be quite different if they tell you that they have had comparable headaches for decades or that they have never had a problem with headaches and this current pain is the worst they have ever experienced. This historical information is every bit as important as laboratory tests or neuroimaging.

A recent report about the value of listening describes the case of a man complaining of a whooshing sound in his left ear. Attention to the patient's description of the sound showed that it was not tinnitus or ringing in the ears but rather the product of abnormal blood flow inside the head. He was found to have multiple cerebral arteriovenous malformations (abnormal tangles of blood vessels connecting arteries and veins). The diagnosis had been delayed because his physicians had assumed that he was reporting a ringing sound.[2]

If I were given a choice that I could rely only on either history, examination, or laboratory tests to make a diagnosis I would certainly choose history. The most important part of the interaction with the patient is the history. The physical exam and lab tests are also important, of course. However, it is remarkable how frequently the diagnosis is apparent based on the history alone. In a study of making diagnoses, it was found that in 76% of cases, the history alone led to the final diagnosis.[3] There are certain situations, of course, in which comprehensive history-taking is not possible until after the immediate needs of the patient are met. In emergency situations such as with chest pain, establishing an intravenous line and taking an EKG are immediately necessary.

The importance of listening is well discussed in *How Doctors Think*, by J. Groopman of Harvard Medical School.[4]

> When you're a student, you're judged by how well you answer questions. But in life, you're judged by how good your questions are.
> —Robert Langer, MIT Chemical Engineer[5]

References

1. Friedland RP, St John JN. Video-game palsy: Distal ulnar neuropathy in a video-game enthusiast. *N Engl J Med*. 1984 Jul 5;311(1):58–9. doi:10.1056/NEJM198407053110121. PMID: 6328304.
2. Bettendorf BA. Listening lessons. *JAMA*. 2023 Mar 21;329(11):883. doi:10.1001/jama.2023.0521. PMID: 36862428.
3. Peterson MC, Holbrook JH, Von Hales D, Smith NL, Staker LV. Contributions of the history, physical examination, and laboratory investigation in making medical diagnoses. *West J Med*. 1992 Feb;156(2):163–5. PMID: 1536065; PMCID: PMC1003190.
4. Groopman J. *How Doctors Think*. Mariner Books; 2008, 179.
5. Gura, T. Robert Langer: Creating things that could change the world. *Science*. 2014 Nov. https://www.science.org/content/article/robert-langer-creating-things-could-change-world

Lesson 6
Be a Good Observer

Being a good observer is essential for critical thinking. Here are some suggestions for being a good observer:

- Don't try to analyze something before you observe it. Observe first, then analyze.
- Record what you observe even if you don't understand—its importance may become apparent later (don't assume that it is not important if you don't understand it).
- Watch out for the many kinds of bias (Lessons 51–53).
- Don't let your observations be clouded because of preconceived ideas.
- Be attentive and observe fully, not while multitasking.
- Use all opportunities to observe (when the patient comes into the room note how they walk and talk, how is their handshake?).
- Does the patient have an odor? What about their clothing?
- Are their shoes of interest (Lesson 2). Uneven wear of the soles may be a sign of gait disturbance and neurological deficit.
- Does the patient make eye contact? Can they hear you?
- How did the patient visit make you feel? If the visit made you sad, consider the possibility that the patient is depressed.

In 1860, Louis Pasteur was studying bacterial growth with a microscope. He smeared a drop of butyric *Vibrios* on a glass slide and saw that the microorganisms at the edges of the smear were immobile, but those at the center were mobile. As reported by the microbiologist Patrice Debre in his biography of Pasteur, "This detail which many observers would have ignored, intrigued Pasteur.... In the drop of water in which the butyric vibrios were swimming, the concentration of oxygen was not everywhere the same. It was high at the periphery and lower in the center of the slide. On the strength of his observation, Pasteur thought that perhaps the quantity of oxygen had a bearing on the motility and the growth of the microorganisms ... he saw that oxygen was harmful to the life of the animalcules. Oxygen, which was believed to be absolutely indispensable to life now marked the frontier for new kind of microorganisms, those that live without air."[1] This was the first evidence that there were life forms that did not require oxygen. Would you have been so perceptive if you had examined the same slide?*

Pasteur went beyond observation to questioning. Observation was the first step to a great discovery. And he didn't stop with the observation: critical thinking led him to ask "Why?"

> If the clinician, as observer, wishes to see things as they really are, he must make a tabular rasa of his mind and proceed without any preconceived notions whatever.
> —Attributed to Jean-Martin Charcot (see also Lesson 54)

Reference

1. Debre P. *Louis Pasteur*. Johns Hopkins University Press; 1998, 109.

---

* Butyric *Vibrios* are anaerobic bacteria that cannot grow in the presence of oxygen.

Lesson 7
Consider the Patient's Experience

In the clinic setting, it is key that you focus on the patient and not on the computer, iPad, or other devices. The patient is trying to tell you what is wrong with them, and you will not get the message if you do not listen and watch. If there is a computer you need to use in the room, you need to be able to look at the computer screen without turning away from the patient.

Be aware of opportunities to express your thoughtfulness and care. If the patient comes in with a heavy coat, help them remove it and place it on a hanger. If you examine their feet and need them to take off their shoes, it is a meaningful expression of care for you to help them put their shoes back on.

It is vitally important that you use words that the patient can understand. This is best evaluated by questioning them after you speak so you have some idea of what they heard you say. It is not acceptable for you or other providers to call patients by their first name unless you are invited to do so.

A visit to the doctor can involve significant stress for the patient and family. It is important to speak slowly and carefully when you provide a diagnosis and treatment plan. Make sure that they understand. It is best to provide information to the patient about what you want them to do in writing. This material should be clear and not confounded with extraneous items that are of little interest. If they leave the visit with several pieces of paper, including a statement of privacy practices, a summary of their vital signs, pages of laboratory tests, and a list of their medications, these extraneous materials may compete for the patient's attention to the key matter—the summary of what you would like them to do.

If the patient has a unilateral neurological deficit, it is best to speak to them on their good side. They may have unilateral neglect (also called *hemi-inattention*), or a unilateral visual deficit which interferes with their ability to pay attention to events coming from that side.[1] Also, patients with diminished awareness may have difficulty projecting their attention into space. If you stand by the side of the bed of a hospitalized patient with cognitive impairment, they may struggle to attend to your words because of the distance separating the two of you. If the patient has hearing or cognitive problems, it may be best to sit near the side of the bed to get closer to the patient's face as you speak.

If the patient is not capable of understanding, do not talk about their condition with their family members in their presence. There have been cases of people recovering from severe neurological damage telling stories about how they could hear what people were saying even though they appeared to be unconscious. Similarly, a patient with dementia may not understand the words spoken in discussion with a family member about nursing home placement, but they may understand the emotional expression and feeling tone of the conversation. It is usually best if the patient and family members can be in the room at the same time, but this may not be advisable if the patient's understanding is impaired.

No one likes to be sick. Family members don't want loved ones to be sick. The doctor doesn't want the patient to be sick. A good doctor must be willing to recognize what is happening and the many ways that denial may influence access to critical information. If you have a man with cognitive difficulties in your office and you wish to know if he is depressed, it is advisable to speak to the patient and his wife both together and in separate rooms. If you question them together, the patient may not give you honest answers for fear of what his spouse's reaction may be.

Similarly, to learn about his level of impairment, it may be best to speak to them together as well as in separate rooms because the spouse may not wish to confront him with disabilities that he may not be willing to acknowledge. This can be done by asking a nurse or medical assistant to ask the spouse to come out to sign paperwork while the patient is being examined or ask the patient to come out to have his blood pressure checked again while you speak to the spouse in the examining room. If you ask the spouse to come to another room for the purpose of talking to her without his presence, the patient may be disturbed.

A similar situation is found in regard to end-of-life care. It is advisable at times to have discussions about prognosis and treatment options both with the patient and spouse together as well as separately.

An informative case of mine was a 72-year-old man who had significant cognitive deficits and a clear diagnosis of Alzheimer's disease. He was a highly successful businessman and was very much the decision-maker of the family. His wife said that the only decision that she ever had to make was what kind of salad dressing to have for dinner. We had a conference with the patient, his wife and two daughters, along with a nurse, social worker, and myself. It was important for him to understand what was going on as best he could because of decisions that needed to be made about financial and legal planning, as well as driving and possession of guns. In the conference, he refused to acknowledge that there was anything wrong with him, angrily rejecting our assertions that he had any memory or other deficits. When the conference was over he grabbed my arm and pulled me into an exam room, closed the door and said "tell me what the **** is the matter with me." He was aware of his impairment but was not able to acknowledge it in the presence of his family. His denial of illness was only expressed when he was with his family. This story emphasizes how it may be important to learn about the patient with family members present as well as with the patient and family members alone.

I saw a 29-year-old patient in a memory disorders clinic complaining of forgetfulness and aggressive behaviors. She had been arrested for public intoxication and did not appreciate my review of the myriad negative effects of alcohol on the brain. She came with her 4-year-old son, and I gave the son a doctor rubber ducky (with a white coat and stethoscope). The patient's resistance to my input was removed by the warmth of this interaction.*

> Regard every suffering person as a human being.
> —**Attributed to Moses Maimonides (1135–1204)**

Reference

1. Friedland RP, Weinstein EA. Hemi-inattention and hemisphere specialization: Introduction and historical review. *Adv Neurol.* 1977;18:1–31. PMID: 411354.

---

* I keep a supply of doctor and nurse rubber duckies in my desk to give to children who come to my office with parents and grandparents. I also have the distinction of having submitted a paper to the journal *Neurology*, "The use of the rubber ducky in the neurological examination." The paper was not published.

Lesson 8
Learn from Your Patients

Learning about your patients as well as learning from your patients helps you at all levels of the doctor–patient interaction. Information you learn about them will help in establishing their diagnosis and making a treatment plan. Showing your interest in the patient also enhances their experience and helps them have confidence in your care. For example, learning that a patient has 10 cats at home may provide a clue to the cause of an infectious disease. If your patient is a historian with a special interest in Italy, for example, you might inquire about their work. The information you obtain might not help you directly in the patient's care, but it will demonstrate your interest in them as a person, which will help the patient have confidence in you. If they have just returned from a trip across an Australian desert, you should ask them about the trip. In this way, you demonstrate interest which helps establish a good connection. And you may learn something about Australian deserts. If they are carrying a book in their hand, ask about the book. You may learn about the book and about the patient's interests.

There is much you can learn from patients that is not only about medicine, of course. It's important to be able to appreciate the lessons that they teach you. Here are four stories illustrating opportunities where I have learned important lessons from my patients.

A 52-year-old man with Down syndrome who also had Alzheimer's disease was cognitively impaired as well as physically disabled. He was always happy to see me. Whenever I came into his room in clinic he would shout "HELLO DOCTOR FRIEDLAND!" in a warm manner, brimming with joy, with a big smile, and give me a hug. He was happy to be there and not worried about all his problems. I found it inspiring and remarkable that he found such happiness in the presence of so much disability. His bright and sunny demeanor toward me reminded me of the importance of one's attitude while I worried about my grants.

A 53-year-old man had cognitive and visual impairment since childhood from an inherited lipid storage disorder. Even though he had pigmentary retinal degeneration and was legally blind, he could see some shapes and colors, but not objects. I was astounded to learn that he painted, and I found that his work was quite beautiful. He was participating in a painting class, and I asked him how he liked it. He smiled and said that he loved the class and said, "I like to learn." His eagerness to pursue learning is a great model for all of us.

I had another patient with Down syndrome who was 56 years old and had Alzheimer's disease. She came in to see me with a very caring couple in their 50s.

I asked them what their relationship to the patient was. They said that the patient grew up in a house next to theirs and was cared for by the patient's mother until the mother's death 20 years ago. At that time the patient had been instructed by her mother to never open the door for anyone. One day the caring couple noted accumulated newspapers on the neighbor's porch, knocked on the door, and found no response. They had the police open the door, who found the daughter inside with the body of her mother who had been dead for several days. There was no person available from her family to take care of the woman. She was adopted by her neighbors and cared for tenderly for more than 20 years. I was profoundly moved by their extraordinary generosity of spirit.

Many years ago, I had a patient with Parkinson's disease who explained how she was personally responsible for the discovery that amantadine is valuable in the treatment of the disease. She was in the early stages of the illness and was seeing neurologist Robert Schwab at the Harvard Medical School in Boston. She received the medication amantadine because of exposure to influenza. (Amantadine is thought to lessen the severity of the viral illness.) She noted an improvement in her Parkinson's signs while on amantadine and told Dr. Schwab, who was not interested and did not believe her observations. She then went off the amantadine and noted that her symptoms became more severe. She went back to Dr. Schwab to convince him of the effect of the medication. Although he was initially hesitant, he was persuaded by her tenacious demonstrations. He subsequently demonstrated its efficacy in a large group of patients in a publication in the *Journal of the American Medical Association*.[1] The patient felt that she deserved credit for her contribution, and I agree.

Reference

1. Schwab RS, England AC Jr, Poskanzer DC, Young RR. Amantadine in the treatment of Parkinson's disease. *JAMA*. 1969 May 19;208(7):1168–70. PMID: 5818715.

Lesson 9
Intellectualization Limits Your Compassion

Intellectualization is a defense mechanism in which thinking is used to avoid feeling. It involves removing oneself from an emotionally stressful event and uses reasoning to prevent awareness of unpleasant or undesirable emotions. This is not an uncommon practice in medicine. Patients with brain diseases are often considered to be amalgams of brain regions and behaviors ascribed to overactive this or underactive that, instead of being a product of the patients' humanity. Of course, there are times when behavior can be attributed to a neurological deficit (such as hallucinations in a complex partial seizure, lack of word understanding in aphasia, and many others). But the humanity of the patient cannot ever be ignored or denied.

Many years ago, I was involved in a research project on unilateral neglect, which is also called *hemi-inattention*.[1,2] In this condition, damage to one of the cerebral hemispheres, often caused by a stroke, causes the patient fail to attend to stimuli from one side. There is a report of an orchestra conductor with unilateral neglect who faced the cellos to his right, ignoring the violin section on his left, and also of a radiologist who neglected to attend to the left side of each X-ray. A story from renowned British neurologist McDonald Critchley reports that a person with left unilateral neglect who is given a pair of gloves and has to put them on will use his neglected left hand to put the glove on the good right hand (because when you put a glove on your right hand you're focusing on your right hand, even though you are using the left hand).

The condition of unilateral neglect is important to recognize because it can interfere with rehabilitation and safety. The presence of neglect can be evaluated by asking the patient to draw something. The degree to which details from both sides of space are represented can be evaluated. A 75-year-old man I saw had a right middle cerebral artery stroke, causing left unilateral neglect. I asked him to draw a tree (see Figure 9.1). Note that the leaves and branches of the tree are mostly found on the right side and not on the left side of the tree. Do you see anything else important in the drawing?

The tree he has drawn is unstable and about to collapse. I do not doubt that this is a representation of the threat to his stability, both literally and figuratively, produced by the stroke. When I showed this figure to other neurologists, I found wide agreement that the distribution of branches and leaves demonstrated left neglect. Few noticed the unstable position of the tree trunk and its symbolic representation—in my view—of the patient's mental state. The drawing demonstrates both the phenomenon of neglect (few leaves and branches on the left side) as well as threat to the patient's survival

Intellectualization Limits Your Compassion

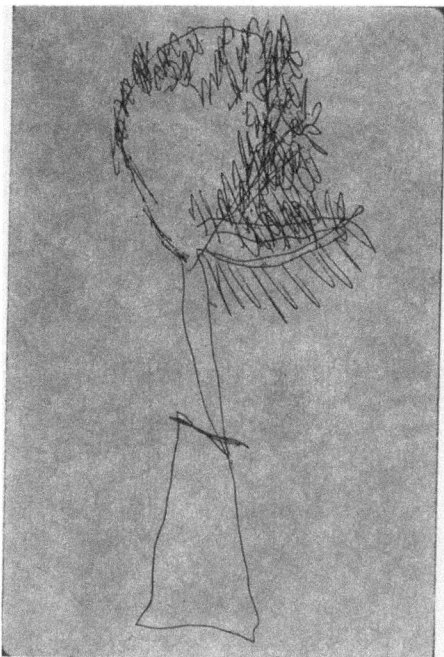

Figure 9.1 Drawing of a tree by a man with a stroke in the right cerebral hemisphere who had neglect of the left side of space.

(the unstable trunk). The neglect is caused by right parietal lobe damage. The fracture of the tree trunk is an expression of the personhood of the patient. The patient does not stop being a person because he's had a stroke.

As a neurology resident I was on rounds in the hospital with other residents and a senior attending. We stopped at the bed of a 45-year-old woman who had been admitted recently for headache. She had had a cerebral angiogram earlier that day and knew we would be telling her what had been found. (This was from the days before CT or MRI scans were available.) The team came into the room and the patient asked the attending if he would like to sit down. She pointed to a chair next to her bed which she had made available for him. He said, "No thank you," put his hand on her shoulder, and said the angiogram showed that she had a brain tumor and that the neurosurgeon would be in to see her shortly. She shuddered and started to cry. Right away he left the room, with the residents following. In the hall, he told us that we should note her "pseudobulbar palsy" caused by dysfunction of the frontal lobes and loss of inhibition. This finding, also called *emotional incontinence*, happens when lesions of the frontal lobes impair the ability to control behavior so that inappropriate crying and laughter may occur. What the attending did not realize was that her tumor had not interfered with her frontal lobe functioning and that she had no signs of inappropriate emotional expression. The reason she was crying was that he just told her she had a brain tumor. I suspect that it made him feel uncomfortable to be in the room with the patient. He violated the basic rules about delivering bad news: the clinician must sit down to demonstrate that the matter is serious and must remain with the patient to answer questions and provide support (Lesson 37). This is an example of intellectualization: he forgot that the patient is a person and not only a brain.

While clinicians need to control their emotions, the emotions must not be entirely suppressed or rejected. Patients need to know that their medical professionals are indeed concerned about their welfare. While it is often stressful caring for sick people, we reject a response of intellectualization and denial. You must allow yourself to have feelings.

Do not hesitate to fully use your most precious instrument, your self.

Most people live in a very restricted circle of their potential being. They make use of a very small portion of their possible consciousness, and of their soul's resources in general, much like a man who, out of his whole organism should get into a habit of using and moving only his little finger.

—William James[3]

References

1. Friedland RP, Weinstein EA. Hemi-inattention and hemisphere specialization: Introduction and historical review. *Adv Neurol.* 1977;18;1–31. PMID: 411354.
2. Bosma MS, Nijboer TCW, Caljouw MAA, Achterberg WP. Impact of visuospatial neglect post-stroke on daily activities, participation and informal caregiver burden: A systematic review. *Ann Phys Rehabil Med.* 2020 Jul;63(4):344–58. doi:10.1016/j.rehab.2019.05.006. Epub 2019 Jun 11. PMID: 31200080.
3. Lutoslawski W. Letter dated 6 May 1906. In *The Letters of William James*. Little, Brown; 1920.

Lesson 10
Key Elements of the Patient Visit
The Interview and Deep Listening

During the patient visit it is key that we observe and listen fully and carefully. When you meet the patient, do they look at you? How are they dressed? Ask open-ended questions and listen. Deep listening is when you listen—*when you just listen*. When you are listening, you are not preparing to speak. After you hear what the patient has to say, you rephrase it back to them to verify that you understand. Recall that most patients have not gone to medical school, so they do not necessarily mean the same thing with the words they use as you do.

The patient must feel free to speak and participate in a dialogue with you.[1]

I saw a 24-year-old patient who had alcohol on his breath and was clearly drunk. I asked him how much alcohol he drank, and he said he didn't drink alcohol. I told him that I could smell alcohol on his breath, and he said, "Oh, that's only beer!" This means that when questioning patients about something such as alcohol intake you must consider the possibility that they don't understand that alcohol includes whiskey, bourbon, wine, beer, and other beverages. The meaning of words is important.

To obtain the social history, you must learn about education, occupation, and recreational activities. It can be important to know not only how many years of education a person has had, but what they studied and what was their level of accomplishment. It is not enough to know, for example, that a patient works for the Army. You must know exactly what they do (a person working for the Army could be involved in producing biological or chemical weapons or have other toxic exposures).

Recreational or nonoccupational activities are the most commonly neglected aspect of the social history. Persons may experience toxic exposures from recreational activities as well as from work, of course. There is a report of a man who enjoyed a hobby of shooting but could not afford the cost of the shooting range. To obtain free time at the shooting range he would sweep up the bullets at the end of the day after they had hit the target and fallen to the ground. His lead poisoning was caused by airborne lead intake through this recreational, not occupational, exposure.[2] Knowing about nonoccupational activities is also a good way to learn about the cognitive capacity of a patient. This can assist in evaluating behavioral deficits and in preparing instructions.

Jewish Torah scribes have been reported with lead poisoning from exposure to an ink produced according to an ancient formula. The scribes control the tip of the brush through moistening on the tongue.[3] Cognitive dysfunction has also been caused by exposure to skin creams containing toxic amounts of bismuth.[4] Women may be exposed to their husbands' occupational hazards through their handling of the laundry. I have often seen workers using agricultural chemicals, including those which are highly neurotoxic, with inadequate precautions.

It is important to learn which medications, supplements, over-the-counter preparations, home remedies, and ethnic preparations the patient takes. If you only ask for medications, the patient will not tell you if they are taking over-the-counter medication such as Tylenol PM, which contains diphenhydramine, which is significantly anticholinergic and can cause memory loss, especially in persons older than 65 years.[5] Women will not tell you that they take birth control pills if you ask them about medications because birth control pills are not considered medicine. Health food products that are widely available may be toxic, but the patient will not tell you about this unless you specifically ask. Vitamins A, B_6, and D may be toxic in high doses. Excessive intake of protein or green tea supplements can cause liver failure.

Sexual history may be important in regard to transmissible diseases. Awareness of the risk of sexually transmissible diseases (HIV, syphilis, gonorrhea, and many others) should not be canceled by a history that does not include potentially hazardous sexual activities. Patients and caregivers may not be aware of the activities of their sexual partners and also may not wish to discuss these activities in the presence of their companions or their doctor. Sexually transmitted diseases are not limited to young persons and should be considered at any age. However, it may not be appropriate to ask questions regarding sexual history in some situations (e.g., I suggest not asking an 80-year-old widow if her recently deceased husband of 50 years had gay lovers because she may not know, may not wish to tell, and may be offended by the question).

A 74-year-old man was seen for paranoid behavior and loss of memory for 1 year. He thought that people were hiding things and "trying to put things over on him." He also complained of an altered sense of smell and taste. He had had a colostomy for cancer of the colon 2 years earlier. His only medication was an oral anti-diabetic agent. Exam showed poor abstraction, judgment, word-finding, and decision-making. Routine blood tests were normal. MRI of the brain showed one small stroke. He worked as a manager of a ball bearing factory, and a panel of tests for heavy metal poisoning was completed because of possible work exposure. It was found that he had a toxic level of the metal bismuth in his blood. Bismuth is known to be an uncommon cause of cognitive impairment. It was subsequently learned that he took a product called bismuth subgallate as a colostomy deodorant. He had not told anyone about this because to him it was not a drug—it was a deodorant, and we had asked him what drugs he was taking. The bismuth product was stopped, and he was markedly improved at 6 months follow-up. He had no further paranoid behavior, complaints of memory loss, or difficulty with executive functioning. His ability to smell and taste returned.[6]

It is critical that healthcare providers are aware of everything being taken, including medications, supplements, vitamins, herbal agents, folk remedies, and other products. A colleague told me of a female patient who was taking a Cambodian herbal remedy for her heart, as well Digoxin from a prescription. Luckily, the physician noticed the oleander picture on the herbal product box and deduced that the patient was digitalis toxic because of double dosing (oleander has toxic cardiac glycosides similar to Digoxin).

It is also important to ask about pets and travel. I saw a man in the hospital in Kyoto, Japan, who had meningoencephalitis caused by *Salmonella*, most likely acquired from his pet turtle. A woman in a mountainous area in California became ill with a high fever after burying her cat who had died of a sudden illness. She was diagnosed with *Yersinia pestis* (the plague) and died despite antibiotic treatment.[7]

An American woman attended a yoga retreat in India and sustained a minor bite by a puppy. She washed the bite and did not think it worthy of further concern. A few weeks later she developed pain in her right arm and became ill with rabies; she subsequently died in the United States.[8] Rabies is approximately 100% fatal after development of symptoms. Patients may not tell you about animal exposures or travel unless you ask!

Although carbon monoxide poisoning is often fatal, low doses can lead to chronic symptoms of cerebral dysfunction.[9] (Carbon monoxide binds to hemoglobin much better than oxygen, causing severe deficiency of oxygen delivery to tissues.) A possible warning of exposure to carbon monoxide at home is the death of pets; because pets are home usually all the time, they are more likely to be exposed. Carbon monoxide poisoning may be caused by poor ventilation of space heaters, as well as waterpipe tobacco smoking.[9]

It is valuable to evaluate the following attributes of the patients' symptoms: duration, timing, quality, severity, and aggravating and relieving factors.

The biggest communication problem is we do not listen to understand. We listen to reply.

—Stephen Covey, American educator[10]

References

1. Groopman J. *How Doctors Think*. Mariner Books; 2008, 179.
2. Novotny T, Cook M, Hughes J, Lee SA. Lead exposure in a firing range. *Am J Public Health*. 1987 Sep;77(9):1225-6. doi:10.2105/ajph.77.9.1225. PMID: 3618861; PMCID: PMC1647000.
3. Cohen N, Modai D, Golik A, Pik A, Weissgarten J, Sigler E, Averbukh Z. An esoteric occupational hazard for lead poisoning. *J Toxicol Clin Toxicol*. 1986;24(1):59-67. doi:10.3109/15563658608990446. PMID: 3084807.
4. Krüger G, Thomas DJ, Weinhardt F, Hoyer S. Disturbed oxidative metabolism in organic brain syndrome caused by bismuth in skin creams. *Lancet*. 1976 Sep 4;1(7984):485-7. doi:10.1016/s0140-6736(76)90786-8. PMID: 74459.
5. Kay GG. The effects of antihistamines on cognition and performance. *J Allergy Clin Immunol*. 2000 Jun;105(6 Pt 2):S622-7. doi:10.1067/mai.2000.106153. PMID: 10856168.

6. Friedland RP, Lerner AJ, Hedera P, Brass EP. Encephalopathy associated with bismuth subgallate therapy. *Clin Neuropharmacol.* 1993 Apr;16(2):173–6. doi:10.1097/00002826-199304000-00010. PMID: 8477413.
7. Gage KL, Dennis DT, Orloski KA, Ettestad P, Brown TL, Reynolds PJ, Pape WJ, Fritz CL, Carter LG, Stein JD. Cases of cat-associated human plague in the Western US, 1977–1998. *Clin Infect Dis.* 2000 Jun;30(6):893–900. doi:10.1086/313804. Epub 2000 Jun 13. PMID: 10852811.
8. Murphy J, Sifri CD, Pruitt R, Hornberger M, Bonds D, Blanton J, Ellison J, Cagnina RE, Enfield KB, Shiferaw M, Gigante C, Condori E, Gruszynski K, Wallace RM. Human Rabies – Virginia, 2017. *MMWR Morb Mortal Wkly Rep.* 2019 Jan 4;67(5152):1410–14. doi:10.15585/mmwr.mm675152a2. PMID: 30605446; PMCID: PMC6334827.
9. Nakamura T, Setsu K, Takahashi T, Miyashita M, Sugiyama N, Washizuka S, Murata S, Hanihara T, Amano N. Chronic exposure to carbon monoxide in two elderly patients using a kotatsu, a traditional Japanese charcoal-based heater. *Psychogeriatrics.* 2016 Sep;16(5):323–6. doi:10.1111/psyg.12164. Epub 2015 PMID: 26551791.
10. Covey S. *The Seven Habits of Highly Effective People.* Simon and Shuster; 2020.

Lesson 11
Words Influence Thought

The great English literary figure of the eighteenth century, Samuel Johnson said, "Language is only the instrument of science, and words are but the sign of ideas." I believe this is seriously incomplete. Language is not only a sign of ideas but also a tool through which ideas are established and transmitted. Words influence how we think. This is true in daily life and politics, as well as in medicine and science.

The influence of words on thought was documented by the work of linguists Edward Sapir (1884–1939) and Benjamin Whorf (1897–1941). They demonstrated that language was not only a way to report experience, but also a mechanism for defining experience. Sapir said, "It is quite an illusion to imagine that one adjusts to reality essentially without the use of language and that language is just an incidental means of solving specific problems of communication ... the real world is, to a large extent, built up on the language habits of the group.... [I]t is a self-contained creative symbolic organization which not only refers to experience ... but actually defines experience."[1]

Whorf came to his ideas through his early work for a fire insurance company. Analyzing hundreds of fires, he found that the words used in many situations were critical influences on the behavior causing the fire. Although the work of Sapir and Whorf on languages of Hopi Indians and Inuit peoples has been challenged, it is important to recognize the influence that words have on thought and action. Their idea that language influences our perceptual and cognitive processes is certainly correct. This is as true in medicine as it is in politics.

The linguist George Lakoff illustrated this in his influential book *Don't Think of an Elephant*.[2] Lakoff illustrates the power of *framing*—to set the terms in which an issue is considered. Framing illustrates that it's often not what you say, it's how you say it.

Examples of the use of word choice to influence understanding are everywhere. In the United States, laws that prevent industry from polluting waterways are referred to as "regulations." The pro-industry political party campaigns for the removal of regulations to liberate manufacturing to be more productive. The word "regulations" has a negative connotation: Who would want to have limitations placed on their activities? Framing the issue with the word "regulations" enhances their position with the public. The more environmentally conscious party will have an unpopular mission if they seek to enhance regulations. I propose that they may further their public appeal if they support "protections" instead of regulations. Furthermore, in the United States, the group wishing to restrict access to abortion call itself "pro-life" and the group supporting abortion rights is "pro-choice." Each group is framing the argument in a manner which supports their view.

An example of the power of words in medicine is the phrase "rule out," which means to eliminate or exclude something from consideration. If I say I have ruled out an infectious cause of a patient's illness, it means that I am absolutely, completely 100% certain that an infectious cause is not responsible for the illness. If I am giving a lecture and ask "Is there an elephant present in this room right now?," I would look around, investigate under the chairs and smell for odors, and, if I don't find an elephant, I can say that I have "ruled out" the possibility that there is an elephant present in the room. In other words, the possibility that there is an elephant present is zero. This is the false-negative rate—the possibility that something is believed to be negative or not found when it is present. A "false-negative" test falsely indicates that a condition is not present. The false-negative rate is rarely zero in medicine. I suggest you never say "rule out" unless you are looking for camels in your cupboard.

There are few situations in medicine where such certainty is possible. Most patients with pneumonia have a fever, but not all. Most patients with an infection in the lining of the heart called endocarditis have blood in the urine, but not all. A patient with a severe headache because of bleeding in the brain who has a spinal tap most commonly has blood in the spinal fluid. However, it is possible for spinal fluid to be normal in patients with intracerebral bleeding.

My fear is that use of the phrase "rule out" implies that there is a greater amount of certainty than is actually present. Rather than consider a condition to be "ruled out" by a test, it is better to say that the test provided evidence that did not confirm the presence of the condition.

In a case of rapidly progressive dementia in a 61-year-old man, a vascular origin was believed by his physicians to have been "ruled out" with a CT scan and a magnetic resonance angiogram. After cerebral angiography, a vascular malformation called an arteriovenous fistula was diagnosed.[3]

Another example of the importance of framing in medicine is presented by American football games in which the quarterback suffers a blow to the head and is reported to have had his "bell rung." The use of the term "bell rung" implies that the sequelae of the event are minor. After all, it is the purpose of a bell to be rung! And the bell could be rung literally 1,000 times a day for 1,000 years and still be working. A report that the player had his "bell rung today" is a linguistic maneuver to divert attention from the fact that his brain suffered a traumatic event. Similarly, motorcycle riders who fall may suffer from "road rash," referring to the skin injury caused by friction when the body strikes the pavement. This is a potentially serious event and calling it a kind of a "rash" limits recognition of its potential severity.

Similarly, an area in which important military events occur is often referred to as the "theater" of war. Referring to a battle as taking place in the theater serves to misrepresent in a devious and immoral manner the true nature of armed conflict. A theater, of course, is not a place where people die. And when a person is killed by his own forces, it is called "friendly fire." It is dangerous to euphemistically imply that war is not brutal and deadly.

A test called a "gold standard" is considered the most accurate test available. I am similarly concerned that the phrase "gold standard" implies that it is perfect, which is not correct. For example, autopsy or biopsy is often considered to be the gold standard test for a medical diagnosis. However, autopsies and biopsies can involve false-positive or false-negative errors just as can any other medical procedure.

Alanine aminotransferase (ALT) and aspartate aminotransferase (AST) are enzymes found in the liver which are elevated in the blood when there is liver damage. Because of this, they are often referred to by clinicians as "liver enzymes." However, both enzymes are also found in muscle and may be elevated in the blood when there is muscle damage. I suggest that improperly calling them "liver enzymes" may obscure the fact that their presence in the blood in high levels may be a sign of muscle and not liver damage.

Another example of the influence of words on thought comes from a $ 3 billion misadventure in space exploration. On April 20, 2023, a Starship rocket of the SpaceX Corporation exploded 4 minutes after takeoff. It was hoped that it would have a 90-minute flight into space. The official report of the event described the outcome as a "rapid unscheduled disassembly." This euphemism is clearly designed to avoid the negative connotations of more common terms, such as "explosion" or "crash."[4] (A *euphemism* is a word or phrase used to avoid an unpleasant or offensive description.)

In February 2023, the guided missile cruiser *Moskva*, of the Russian Navy, which was one of the lead ships of Russia's actions in the Black Sea and the most powerful warship in the region, was sunk by Ukrainian missiles. At the time of the attack Russian radio reported that the ship was "not floating properly." It was soon revealed that this was a euphemism for "sunk."

Euphemisms have often been used by corporations to presumably lessen the stress of termination. Some euphemistic phrases describing firing include involuntary separation from payroll, restructuring, career change opportunity, involuntary severance, career transition program, reduction in force, elimination of employment security, and right-sizing the bank.

A *metaphor* is another figure of speech of interest to us. A metaphor is when a name or phrase is "transferred to an object or action different from, but analogous to, that to which it is literally applicable" (Oxford English Dictionary). If you say that someone is a "shining star" you did not actually mean that she is a celestial body. All words are metaphors in that they are not the same thing as the object or action they represent.

Metaphors are widely used in poetry and other forms of literature. They are also used widely in medicine and science, and the metaphors we choose can have powerful impact on our understanding. On a deeper level, the use of metaphor can blind us to the objective reality of the world. If today is Monday, it is natural to think that it is similar to the Mondays we have had in the past and also similar to the Mondays we will have in the future. And this may be partly correct, as you may have certain activities you do on Mondays that you don't do on other days. That is, the use of the word

"Monday" has value. However, we should be aware that the name "Monday" hides the fact that every day is different from every other day. Even though we call it Monday, it is not a day which has never happened before and which will never happen again.

It is not possible or desirable to live without use of metaphor because metaphor enriches our expressive opportunities. Rather, we should learn to understand how the words we choose influence our understanding and how we comprehend the world. It is critical in medicine for words to mean what they say.

George Lakoff (1941-): A Person to Know

Lakoff is an American philosopher, linguist, and cognitive scientist. He has championed the idea that thought is strongly influenced by the metaphors that are used. His 2004 book *Don't Think of an Elephant* shows the important influence of framing for thought. His work has important implications for medicine and science.[2]

> Our ordinary conceptual system, in terms of which we both think and act, is fundamentally metaphorical in nature.
>
> —George Lakoff[5]

> There is something that causes me the greatest difficulty and continues to do so without relief: unspeakably more depends on what things are called than on what they are.
>
> —Friedrich Nietzsche (1844–1900) German philosopher[6]

References

1. Weinstein EA. Symbolization and the Sapir Whorf hypothesis. *Contemporary Psychoanalysis.* 1973;9:2.
2. Lakoff G. *Don't Think of an Elephant!: Know Your Values and Frame the Debate.* Chelsea Green Publishing; 2014.
3. Rizzo AC. Clinical reasoning: Rapidly progressive thalamic dementia. *Neurology.* 2021 Feb;96(5):e809–e813. doi:10.1212/WNL.0000000000011161.
4. Victor D, Chang K. Starship exploded, but SpaceX had reason to pop champagne anyway. *New York Times.* Apr 20, 2023.
5. George L, Johnson M. *Metaphors We Live By.* University of Chicago Press; 1980.
6. Nietzsche F. *The Gay Science* (1882). Vintage; 1974.

Lesson 12
The Physical Exam

It is advisable to perform the physical exam in a certain consistent order. For example, if you see a patient who complains of weakness of the left foot, do not begin the exam with the feet. They may have leukemia, and that diagnosis may be suggested by the presence of retinal hemorrhages. If you go immediately to examine the foot, you may forget to examine the eyes. A patient with chronic abdominal pain may have lymphoma, and if you go immediately to the abdominal exam you may forget to examine the lymph nodes in the neck.

The mental status exam is an important part of the patient encounter. It is critical to know if the patient is fully oriented and if they are aware of what's happening. If you prescribe medications, it is always critical for you to know if they can understand your instructions.

Make sure that you examine all of the patient. This will require you to ask them to take their clothes off. A person with a high fever who also has pink, pinprick-sized lesions and larger, purple, bruise-like markings may have meningococcal meningitis, a diagnosis which requires great urgency. These spots may be on the back and may be missed if the patient is not undressed. Do the fingernails show evidence of endocarditis (splinter hemorrhages)? Is there an abnormalty of the patient's hair?

A man came to the emergency room with acute chest pain in the left upper chest. He was examined by the emergency room doctor and found to have normal heart sounds, a normal EKG, and normal cardiac enzymes. Because of consideration of a myocardial infarction, he was sent to the ICU. There his shirt was removed and it was found that he had a dislocated shoulder. A distinguished neurologist I know failed his pediatric neurology board examination because he did not take off the baby's diaper during the exam.

Many years ago, I saw a patient in the emergency room in a hospital in Chinatown, New York City, who had been stabbed in the abdomen. I urgently started intravenous fluids and arranged for an ambulance to take him to Bellevue Hospital. When we arrived, he was moved off a stretcher on to the emergency room bed and we noticed that he was also stabbed in the back. I was not aware of that because I had not looked.

A 95-year-old man who was the father of a friend had chest pain and called for emergency assistance. He was brought to the emergency room by ambulance and was examined by the physician. Intravenous fluids were started and EKG, chest X-ray, lab tests, and vital signs were normal. The cause of his complaint was unclear, and he was brought to the ICU. A nurse practitioner took a brief history and did one other thing to reveal the diagnosis. She removed his shirt and saw an acute rash, indicative of a herpes zoster (shingles) infection. This painful neuronal condition had not been observed because no one had removed his shirt. The emergency room physician had examined his heart and lungs through his shirt, which is not recommended. (The man was given appropriate treatment for herpes zoster, was sent home, and lived to be 108.)

I saw a patient who had status epilepticus in which the only sign was a jerking movement of one toe because the major motor manifestations of the seizures had become exhausted with time and the only evidence of the condition that remained was the jerking of the toe. This would not have been noted if the patients' blanket had not been removed.

It is best to always examine the patient from the same side. It is generally recommended that the right side is better, because it allows your right hand to palpate the liver. If you do it always on the same side, you will obtain more practice than if you alternate right and left. At times, in the hospital, you may need to move the bed and chairs around to access the patient on the right side. It is often worthwhile to do so.

> Get the patient in a good light. Use your five senses. We miss more by not seeing than we do by not knowing. Always examine the back. Observe, record, tabulate, communicate.
>
> —William Osler[1]

Reference

1. Osler W. *The Evolution of Modern Medicine*. Kessinger; 2004, 71. ISBN 1-4191-6153-91.

Lesson 13
Touch Is Important

Physical touch is a powerful mode of communication and a force for healing. Research has shown the potent influence of touch on feeling state and illness.[1] There is a long history of prohibition of touch between physician and patient based on sexualization of touch and erroneous teachings in psychiatry. American psychiatrist Karl Menninger (1898–1990) said that physical contact with the patient is "evidence of incompetence or criminal ruthlessness of the analyst." The American psychoanalyst Lewis Wolberg said "Physical contact with the patient is absolutely a taboo since it may mobilize sexual feelings in the patient and the therapist and bring forth violent outbursts of anger."[2] These views should be considered obsolete.

Touch is an important part of the neurological examination, and the exam is a necessary part of the medical encounter. It is not possible to know how much resistance to passive motion is present without holding the hand and moving the arm and forearm. When I ask a patient to get up so I can see how they walk, I may offer them my hand to help them rise from the chair. Shaking the patient's hand when you meet them is a small but valuable demonstration of care. The nature of the patient's grip during a handshake can also impart information about the skin, motor function, and emotional state. Shaking a patient's hand when you are done is also valuable because it provides a nonverbal cue indicating that the consultation is over. This is a good way for the patient to understand that they need to ask any remaining questions right away, before the physician has gone. It is also valuable to find ways to touch patients who are seen in the hospital. This can be done with shaking hands, of course, but also holding their feet as part of the examination. If there is any question about the possible misunderstanding of touch, the exam can be done with a chaperone or a nurse or aide present.

The physician–patient partnership works best when the humanity of both participants is allowed to flourish. Touching the patient may be one way in which this shared humanity can be expressed. At times there is not much that can be said in response to suffering. Being there with the patient and caregiver in silence can be a powerful way to care. **Silence is a powerful force that must be respected.**

Many of the problems we face cannot be fixed through drugs, surgery, or other means. Sometimes the best we can do is be there, bear witness, and be silent. As noted by neurologist Vladimir Hachinski in a paper "Poets as Guides in Medicine, Research, and Life," "our most grateful patients are not the ones we do the most for, that is expected from modern medicine, but the ones we can do the least for, whom we offer our deeply felt empathy or love."[3]

Empathy, presence, and nonabandonment require more of the physician as a person than as a scientist.

—M. Bretscher, British biologist[4]

There are problems that are entirely human and existential and are not amenable to quick solution by technology.... Much of what we are asking is outside the scope of medicine.... Sometimes what is needed is to bear witness or to be silent.

—Carlos Gomez, American palliative care physician[5]

References

1. Zur O. To touch or not to touch: Exploring prohibition on touch in psychotherapy and counseling and the ethical considerations of touch. https://www.zurinstitute.com/resources/touch-in-therapy. Accessed May 29, 2020.
2. Wolberg LR. *The Technique of Psychotherapy* (2nd ed.). Grune & Stratton; 1967, 2.
3. Hachinski V. Poets as guides in medicine, research, and life. *Neurology*. 2023 Oct 17;101(16):721–2. doi:10.1212/WNL.0000000000207582. Epub 2023 Jul 25. PMID: 37491323; PMCID: PMC10585671.
4. Bretscher ME, Creagan ET. Understanding suffering: What palliative medicine teaches us. *Mayo Clin Proc*. 1997;72(8):785–7.
5. Gomez C. Re-examining the Dutch experience with physician-assisted suicide. Presented at the 11th International Congress on Care of the Terminally Ill. Quebec, Montreal; 1996.

Lesson 14
Be Prepared for the Unexpected

There is no technology which is not capable of error. If you get a laboratory result which is significantly abnormal and unexpected, it is worth considering if the result is an error. It may be desirable to repeat the test to see if the same result is obtained.

More than 30–40% of medications are not taken in the correct manner. Poor compliance with medications is estimated to take the lives of more than 100,000 Americans every year. The risk of poor compliance is up to 100% if the patient is taking 10 medications. It is best if all the things that the patient is taking are brought in for examination by the medical care team, and it is important that all medications are reviewed at each visit. This review should include the dose, the frequency, and the need to take with or without food. Supplements, vitamins, and herbal and ethnic remedies all need to be considered. If you only ask for medications, the patient will not tell you that they are taking a toxic amount of vitamin D, for example.

The health of the patient commonly suffers when they do not take their medications in the right way. A less common but significant problem is that the incorrect medications may have been placed in the bottle. I am aware of a patient with cognitive impairment who was prescribed 0.5 mg of haloperidol once a day for agitation. He did poorly and the doctor increased the dose to three times a day; the patient died. It was revealed that the pharmacist had given him 5.0 mg pills of the drug, instead of 0.5 milligram pills. Another case involved a woman who was given an anticoagulant instead of an antidepressant. It's not surprising that she died of bleeding. Although this is certainly an uncommon problem, it requires consideration and awareness.

As a resident at Mount Sinai Hospital in New York City, I was told the story of a patient with complex cognitive problems and neuropathy who was being poisoned with arsenic by his wife. In Lesson 32. I discuss the story of a neurologist killed by her husband with cyanide.[1] The possibility that the family does not have the best interests of the patient in mind should be considered.

While I was a resident, a patient suffered a grievous error made in the performance of a carotid angiogram. The procedure involved placing a catheter in the internal carotid artery, infusing a dye, and recording the passage of the dye through the brain. Before the procedure began, two identical basins were prepared, one containing alcohol for cleaning the skin and the other containing the dye. Tragically, the person performing the angiogram injected the alcohol instead of the dye into the carotid artery, which was rapidly fatal. The two liquids were confused because of their similar color. Following this disaster, Betadine, which is red, was adopted for skin cleaning.

Many of the scientific advances discussed in this book depended on the ability of the investigator to observe what happened and to welcome the opportunity to deal with unexpected results. There are also scientists, of course, who do not want unexpected results. It may be that they are so attached to their hypotheses that anything unexpected is rejected as false. It may also be that they only do research that is predictable. For example, I worked with someone whose favorite kind of study was the effect of aging on X in the rat (X could be blood flow, metabolism, or any number of other subjects). This individual criticized a proposed project of mine by saying that I did not know what would be found. This attitude toward investigation is unfortunate and disturbing. The beauty of science is its ability to allow for new learning. If an investigation does not involve new learning, it's not worth doing.*

A magnificent account of the importance of appreciation of unexpected results is the book *Introduction to Experimental Medicine*, by Claude Bernard (1865).[2]

> The search for knowledge is an endless process and one can never know how it is going to turn out. Unpredictability is in the nature of the scientific enterprise. If what is to be found is really new, then it is by definition unknown in advance. There is no way of telling where a particular line of research will lead. This is why it is not possible to select some parts of science and to reject others.... Either you have science or you don't have it. And if you have it you cannot take only what you like. You have to accept as well the unexpected and disturbing results.
> —Max Perutz (1914–2002), British molecular biologist, winner of the 1962 Nobel Prize in Chemistry for uncovering the structures of myoglobin and hemoglobin[3]

Claude Bernard (1813–1878): A Person to Know

Bernard was a French physiologist and originator of the term *"milieu interieur,"* which later became *homeostasis*. He discovered the role of the liver in storing glucose as glycogen, and he disclosed the role of the pancreas in digestion. He demonstrated the importance of animal research and careful experimentation. He was a friend of Louis Pasteur and helped foster the use of scientific methods in medicine.

References

1. Ward P. *Death by Cyanide: The Murder of Dr. Autumn Klein*. ForeEdge; 2016.
2. Bernard C. *An Introduction to the Study of Experimental Medicine*. Dover Books; 1927.
3. Perutz MF. *I Wish I'd Made You Angry Earlier: Essays on Science, Scientists, and Humanity*. Cold Spring Harbor Lab Press; 2002.

---

* Research that provides replication of previous results is new learning.

SECTION II
DIAGNOSIS AND EVALUATION

Lesson 15
The Fundamental Three-Step Approach to Diagnosis

If you see a patient in the emergency room who has been struck by an arrow that is embedded in his neck, you should undoubtedly focus your attention on the wound and, of course, the patient's airway, breathing, and circulation. When the situation is not as emergently critical as that, you have time to follow a three-step approach. This approach is valuable for all aspects of medical care.

First, signs and symptoms. Evaluate the nature of the signs and symptoms. Ask open-ended questions and listen. Symptoms are what the patient tells you is wrong (what are they experiencing?). Signs are what you have learned with the physical examination. It is critical to listen to understand, not listen to reply. Be sure to understand what the patient means when she speaks. If they say dizzy, they may mean weak, and if they say weak, they may mean dizzy (or something else entirely). Assess the patient through the physical examination to determine the meaning of the symptoms and signs. If a patient complains of slurred speech, is it because of a problem with language or a difficulty with coordination of the tongue, lips, and throat? Are the problems getting worse or better? What are the associated symptoms or signs? Where precisely are the symptoms located? Can they point them out with one finger? What makes them better, and what makes them worse?

When you are early in the evaluation of the patient try not to jump ahead and determine the localization of the problem or the cause of the problem before you have figured out what the problem is.

It is hard to exaggerate the importance of the history of the present illness. The nature in which symptoms appear often provides physicians with all the information needed to select diagnostic possibilities and eliminate others. Consider this scenario: a 50-year-old woman presents with numbness and weakness in the left leg and white matter damage in the cerebrum on the right on MRI imaging. The differential diagnosis will be influenced by knowing if this event is the only event of neurological dysfunction she has ever had. If you learn, on the other hand, that she had a period of blurred vision in her right eye that lasted 2 weeks at the age of 28 the possibility of multiple sclerosis will be suggested.

If a patient presents with fatigue, there are many possible causes. If they also have muscle weakness, depression, difficulty controlling their emotions, memory loss, headache, weight gain, change in the shape of the face, stretch marks on the breasts and abdomen, and easy bruising, Cushing's syndrome should be suspected.*

Second, localization. After you have evaluated the symptoms and signs consider which part of the body is involved. If there is difficulty speaking, is it caused by a lesion in the mouth, pharynx, or neck? Is it caused by a brain lesion affecting the strength and coordination of the muscles involved in speech? Or is it aphasia (a brain lesion affecting the production and understanding of speech)? If there was a neurological problem, what anatomical localization would be most likely? Is it caused by a problem in the head, and, if so, what side and what part of the brain or cranial nerves? If there is weakness in one foot, is it likely to be caused by a lesion in muscle, peripheral nerves, nerve roots, the spinal cord, brainstem, cerebral hemisphere, or cortex? If there is flank pain, is it coming from the muscles, or is it of deeper origin (kidneys?). Again, try not to consider etiology until you have considered the localization.

Third, etiology. Finally, in consideration of the signs and symptoms and likely localization, what etiology (cause) is most probable? It is best to consider the most probable cause or causes, but don't lose awareness of others. It is valuable to use the VITAMINS ABCD mnemonic described in the next lesson to consider the classes of etiologies that may be responsible. It is not uncommon that consideration of one diagnosis obscures the possibilities of others. Routine use of the VITAMINS ABCD mnemonic helps to remind us of the full range of possibilities. Application of the mnemonic may only take a few minutes.

Harvey Cushing (1869–1939): A Person to Know

Cushing was an American neurosurgeon and pathologist who was the first surgeon to concentrate on the brain. He also was the first to describe Cushing's disease, which is associated with excessive secretion of adrenocorticotropic hormone (ACTH) from the anterior pituitary. He developed many of the techniques used today for surgery on the brain. His biography of Sir William Osler won a Pulitzer Prize (1926).[1] Cushing also advanced methods for the measurement and recording of blood pressure in the operating room.

Reference

1. Cushing H. *The Life of Sir William Osler.* Gryphon Editions; 1993.

---

* Cushing's syndrome is a hormonal disorder which occurs when there is excessive cortisol secretion.

Lesson 16
A Mnemonic for Etiologies, VITAMINS ABCD

V   Vascular
I   Infectious/Inflammatory
T   Toxic/Traumatic
A   Autoimmune
M   Metabolic
I   Inherited/Iatrogenic
N   Neoplastic
S   Seizures
A   Allergic
B   Behavioral
C   Congenital
D   Degenerative

It is wise to realize the difference between etiology and pathogenesis. *Etiology* is the cause and *pathogenesis* is the process by which the disease develops and sustains itself. The etiology of paralytic poliomyelitis is the poliovirus. The pathogenesis of paralytic poliomyelitis disease is the death of motor neurons caused by the virus. We know the etiology of Huntington's disease: the disease is caused by an abnormally high number of trinucleotide repeats on the huntigtin gene on chromosome 4. We do not yet understand the pathogenesis of the disease because we don't know why the high number of trinucleotide repeats make people sick. The pathogenesis of Alzheimer's disease involves abnormally folded proteins and neuroinflammation in a complex series of events. The etiology of the disease in the 99% of cases that are not caused by an autosomal dominant mutation remains unknown.

Remember also that pathology is not pathogenesis.[1] Imagine the scenario of Berlin in May 1945. The city had been heavily bombed and most buildings were destroyed. A comprehensive analysis of what was wrong in the city (the pathology) would not help in understanding the processes that resulted in the bombing (the pathophysiology). Similarly, in Parkinson's disease, there are deposits of fibrillar alpha synuclein deposits in neurons in the midbrain and other regions. That is an important aspect of the pathology of the disease but has not yet helped us understand the pathophysiology of the illness.

You will often see patients who appear to have a clearly defined condition with a certain etiology. It is always helpful to consider other possible etiologies which may not be as obvious. For example, a patient with a progressive neurological deficit with swelling in one part of the brain may have a brain tumor. The prospect that the lesion is infectious should not be ignored (e.g., a brain abscess). A person with diarrhea may have an intestinal infection. The chance that it is toxic is also worth considering. Vertigo, the feeling that you or the environment is moving when it is not, may be caused by diseases of the inner ear, as well as by arrythmia (abnormal heart rhythm), hypotension, brain tumor, and stroke. The possibility that vertigo can also be caused by vitamin deficiency should also be considered, especially B_{12} and B_1 (thiamine).

A teacher of mine in New York City was an orthodox Jew who came down with headaches, fever, weakness, and muscle pain. After a difficult and slow differential diagnosis, it was discovered that he had trichinosis (an infection with the worm *Trichinella*). He did not eat pork, bear, or cougar (three sources of the parasite). It was eventually established that he had gone to a butcher shop for ground beef and ate it raw (this is a popular dish in French cuisine). The organism causing trichinosis cannot be found in beef. The butcher had illegally used the same meat grinder for pork followed by beef, thus causing his infection. I propose that the use of the VITAMINS ABCD algorithm may have provided a faster diagnosis in this case.

The possibility that disorders of older persons may be genetic is often neglected. Seizures may have unusual presentations which are not obviously epileptic, such as speech arrest, laughing, hallucinations, or weakness.

The use of VITAMINS ABCD will be helpful to increase your consideration of potential etiologies that are not readily evident. **You will not make a diagnosis if you don't think of it.** VITAMINS ABCD will help you to widen your diagnostic perspective.[2,3]

References

1. Espay AJ, Okun MS. Abandoning the proteinopathy paradigm in Parkinson disease. *JAMA Neurol.* 2023 Feb 1;80(2):123–4. doi:10.1001/jamaneurol.2022.4193. PMID: 36441542.
2. Zabidi-Hussin ZA. Practical way of creating differential diagnoses through an expanded VITAMINSABCDEK mnemonic. *Adv Med Educ Pract.* 2016 Apr 22;7:247–8. doi:10.2147/AMEP.S106507. PMID: 27217805; PMCID: PMC4853007.
3. Gawande A. *The Check List Manifesto.* Henry Holt; 2009.

Lesson 17
Investigations

Information is valuable. But is all information of value? Is it possible to have too much information? Information can be helpful or harmful, depending on the situation, and excessive information can be dangerous. **Data are useless unless translated into information.**

Investigations should be considered in regard to the risk-benefit ratio. A complete blood count is of essentially no risk, is low cost, and can often be important. A spinal tap is also very low risk and often is of great value. A low-risk procedure may be advisable even if the potential benefit is not highly probable. A high-risk procedure should only be performed if the prospect for benefit is significant.

In considering the risk-benefit ratio, it is worthwhile to anticipate what will be the effect of the investigation. If it may reveal information that will change the patient's management, then it may be advised. If it is clear that the result will not affect management or outcome, then it may not be indicated.

What about predictive tests? **The important standard is always what difference it will make to the patient.** Discovery of a precancerous lesion in the colon via colonoscopy may save someone's life. A positron emission tomography (PET) scan may show amyloid beta protein deposits in the brain of a cognitively healthy 75-year-old person. This would mean that her risk of developing Alzheimer's disease is increased. However, we cannot say at which age dementia will develop and if she will live long enough for that to happen. It may be likely that she will die with the deposits in the brain without developing cognitive impairment. The critical factor is that there is currently no disease-modifying therapy available to alter the course of the illness.[1] This is why it is not recommended to perform amyloid beta protein PET scans in cognitively unimpaired persons.

Genetic testing may help to plan ways to serially monitor a patient for development of a disease that is preventable or treatable. Discovery of a genetic finding may also help identify options for participation in clinical trials. If there is no effective intervention available, genetic testing for risk factor genes may cause unnecessary worry and concern.

For example, I know of two health-conscious university professors who had themselves tested for the apolipoprotein E e4 gene (allele), which confers a high risk of Alzheimer's disease (compared to people without the e4 allele).[2] They were asymptomatic and found that they each had one copy of the risk gene, thus increasing their risk by a factor of about 4 times. Their 28-year-old daughter, also health-conscious and asymptomatic, had herself tested and found that she unfortunately had two copies of the risk gene, which increases her risk of having the disease by a factor of about 10. However, it is still possible for all of them to reach late ages without getting the disease. It is also possible for people without the gene to get the disease.[1,2]

It is widely stated that information about genetic risk can help people to follow certain lifestyle behaviors, such as a low saturated fat diet, physical and mental exercise, avoidance of head injury and environmental toxins, and other factors.[1] Nevertheless, it is advisable to follow these lifestyle practices even if you do not have a certain gene, because you can still get Alzheimer's disease without having the gene. I am concerned that the 28-year-old woman may worry about this enhanced risk for the next 60 or so years, and, if she is cognitively unimpaired at the age of 88, she can conclude that she didn't have to worry about it for the past 60 years. The situation would be different if there was a curative treatment that could be applied based on knowledge of the genetic risk. But this is not presently the case.

It is best for decisions about genetic testing to be made with the advice of a genetic counselor. Genetic risks are complex factors that can be difficult to comprehend.

Imaging procedures have also been developed to detect early stages of disease. Imaging of the body can be very rewarding, of course. However, the radiation exposure involved in X-rays and CT scans needs to be considered in comparison to the benefit to be obtained. Imaging may reveal abnormalities that require further evaluation, which may be hazardous, even though the finding turns out to be benign (Lesson 20). The use of artificial intelligence systems for analysis of X-rays, CT and MRI scans, and other imaging methods will be helpful. But interpreting the results of computer-based systems will require appropriate expertise.

References

1. Friedland RP. *Unaging: The Four Factors That Impact How You Age*. Cambridge University Press; 2022.
2. Andrews SJ, Renton AE, Fulton-Howard B, Podlesny-Drabiniok A, Marcora E, Goate AM. The complex genetic architecture of Alzheimer's disease: Novel insights and future directions. *EBioMedicine*. 2023 Apr;90:104511. doi:10.1016/j.ebiom.2023.104511. Epub 2023 Mar 10. PMID: 36907103; PMCID: PMC10024184.

Lesson 18
Don't Be Afraid To Say You Don't Know

Awareness that you don't know something is a pivotal step toward understanding. The first stage in the search for knowledge must be the comprehension of your current state of knowledge. What is it you know, and what is it that you don't know? How do you know that your current knowledge is reliable? Do you know what you know now because of what somebody told you, because of what you read about, or because of something that you learned for yourself? These questions apply equally to clinical or scientific matters.

Believing that you have identified the patient's diagnosis may prevent you from pursuing other measures that would uncover the correct diagnosis. Being aware that you don't know opens wide the possibilities. This is a difficult problem in medicine because physicians tend to be relatively intellectual and confident in their own reasoning abilities.

Many persons in medicine and science find it difficult to appreciate the fact that they may be ignorant of many things. In my training, I had one chief, Morris B. Bender, who often said that he didn't know what was happening with the patient, even though he had enormous clinical experience. He would say, "I'm just a boy, I don't know. It's a puzzlement." (He was the president of the American Neurological Association, 1972–1973.) I had another teacher during my training who would never admit that he didn't know a patient's diagnosis. He was often wrong, but never in doubt.

One story illustrates the pervasive need for physicians to be certain. I heard a lecture by a distinguished neuro-ophthalmologist about temporal arteritis (a form of giant cell vasculitis). He said that all cases had onset at the age of 55 or later. At the end of the lecture, a physician asked him about a patient with all the features of temporal arteritis who happened to have onset at the age of 53. When the lecturer said that this patient could not possibly have temporal arteritis, he was asked why and the speaker said that the patient was too young. Clearly the speaker had undue confidence in his assumed knowledge.

The problem of inappropriate confidence in incorrect beliefs is an enormous issue in the history of medicine and science. A great value in the study of history is the understanding that our ancestors where just like us. We may say today that we can't believe that leeches were prescribed widely for many problems. Similar statements will be made about us in the future. An enormous cause of the erroneous beliefs of the past concerning human health was not only that they didn't know, but that they didn't know that they didn't know.

Being aware of your ignorance is difficult, especially since our education is devoted to learning what is considered to be "facts." In the earlier years of my education, I learned these facts about the body: every neuron had one neurotransmitter, the animal most closely linked by evolution to humans is the gorilla, the genes of one animal could not possibly be moved to another, human genes cannot be changed, the only mechanism of genetic transmission from one generation to another involved changes in the nucleotide sequence, dementia in old age is caused by aging alone, and Alzheimer's disease was caused by "hardening of the arteries in the neck." All of these "facts" have been proved wrong.

False knowledge is hazardous. Lack of awareness of ignorance diminishes exploration and investigation. For decades it was "known" that peptic ulcers were caused by excessive acid and needed to be treated with restrictive bland diets (the Sippy Diet). The idea, which won the Nobel Prize in Physiology or Medicine for Marshall and Warren, that gastric bacteria were causative was not accepted because it contradicted the "fact" that bacteria could not grow in the stomach (they can; Lesson 48).[1]

In another example, we know that two copies of the apolipoprotein E epsilon 4 gene is associated with a higher risk of Alzheimer's disease. Many physicians would say that a person with two copies of the gene who had dementia had the disease because of the gene.[2] However, people who have two copies of the gene can have a long life and not get dementia. This says to me that there must be something else involved. If we assume that the causation in these cases is entirely genetic, our search for other critical factors is inhibited.

You may feel stupid at times. That's OK. It is helpful to recognize that medical and scientific problems can be intrinsically hard. Research problems are by their very nature without answers. If we knew clearly what was happening, we wouldn't have to do research about it. It is important to recognize that research questions are often difficult. If we knew the answer already it wouldn't be research!

Oliver Wendel Holmes (1841–1935) American legal scholar and jurist put it well when he said, "Science is the topography of ignorance."

This point of view is discussed in a one-page paper, "The importance of stupidity in scientific research," by cell biologist Martin Schwartz. He says "The scope of things we don't know is infinite.... One of the beautiful things about science is that it allows us to bumble along, getting it wrong time after time and feel perfectly fine as long as we learn something each time ... the more comfortable we become with being stupid the deeper we will wade into the unknown and the more likely we are to make big discoveries."[3]

Intellectual humility involves the recognition that we don't know everything and that our current views may be in error. This is linked to learning, educational achievement, and critical thinking as intellectual humility enhances comprehension of varying perspectives. According to psychologist Tenelle Porter, "intellectual humility can really help us listen to those who don't have the same ways of knowing as we do." Humility is also a key factor in the success of collaborations.[4]

The first step of being aware of our ignorance is to learn to admit to yourself and to others when you don't know. And allow your ignorance to be a stimulus to your clinical and scientific work.

> Thoroughly conscious ignorance is the prelude to every real advance in science.
> —**James Clerk Maxwell (1831–1879), Scottish scientist, responsible for the classical theory of electromagnetism**

> To be Humane we must ever be ready to pronounce that wise, ingenious and modest statement, "I do not know."
> —**Galileo (1564–1642)**

References

1. Nobel Prize Organization. Barry Marshall Nobel lecture. 2005. https://www.nobelprize.org/prizes/medicine/2005/marshall/lecture/
2. Andrews SJ, Renton AE, Fulton-Howard B, Podlesny-Drabiniok A, Marcora E, Goate AM. The complex genetic architecture of Alzheimer's disease: Novel insights and future directions. *EBioMedicine*. 2023 Apr;90:104511. doi:10.1016/j.ebiom.2023.104511. Epub 2023 Mar 10. PMID: 36907103; PMCID: PMC10024184.
3. Schwartz MA. The importance of stupidity in scientific research. *J Cell Sci*. 2008 Jun 1;121(11):1771. doi:10.1242/jcs.033340. PMID: 18492790.
4. Porter T. Blog. https://transformativefuturelearning.home.blog/blog-feed. Accessed Nov 2, 2023.

Lesson 19
Information Toxicity

The brain is capable of processing only a certain amount of information at a time. There is a danger that excessive data will have negative effects on performance, and "information toxicity" can result if the attentional capacity is exceeded. Excessive data make it hard to appreciate what is important.

Imagine an airplane cockpit approaching a runway; the plane is about to land in a heavy rain with strong winds. Will the copilot tell the captain "I'd like you to know, captain, that we have 178 passengers, 99 women, 51 men and 28 children. Also, the first-class cabin passengers did not eat all of their meals, so, if you like, after we land, you can have your choice of steak or fish." Of course, landing the plane requires fast and accurate decision-making. Many decisions made in medicine do not require such speed. However, the competition for attention and awareness exists in the clinic just as it does in the cockpit. If I get 10 pages of lab tests about a new patient, I would prefer not to be informed about irrelevant information (Was the blood pressure taken in the left or right arm? What kind of blood pressure cuff was used? Who took the blood pressure? What is the patient's body surface area?). These items are rarely important, and their presence in the electronic health record makes it more difficult for me to be aware of what's happening.

To avoid information toxicity, we should be clear that whatever data we collect is both valid and relevant. Mathematician Francis Dalton famously said, "whenever you can, count." This is generally good advice. If I have a patient who cannot reverse a five-letter word, I may see if they can reverse a four-letter word to better quantify the deficit. However, it is advisable to avoid carefully quantifying things which are not reliable (*reliable* means consistently high quality and giving the same answer on repeated trials). Computer programs can do all sorts of powerful statistical analyses that are a waste of time if the data are meaningless. Don't report the data with extreme precision which is not supported by the method of data collection. For example, body mass index (BMI) is a person's weight in kilograms divided by the square of height in meters. If a patient's BMI is recorded as 38.43, this indicates that she is obese. It is not necessary or wise to remember or record all four of these numbers! The 0.03 BMI units has no meaning whatsoever (perhaps it is the result of eating two cookies). Such unnecessary precision should not be included in electronic health records, and we should not pay attention to data which has no meaning. Don't report data with more detail than needed.

In the United States, there is enormous pressure to enhance the documentation of every outpatient visit in order to bill at a higher level. Therefore, the record may include copies of lab tests and other procedures, and an outpatient visit may end up being more than 10 pages long, making it difficult to know what is actually happening.

More information is not always better. A randomized multicenter clinical trial in four ICUs of adults requiring a week of mechanical ventilation examined the effect of structured family meetings and emotional support led by palliative care specialists. It was found that the intervention *increased* anxiety and posttraumatic stress disorder (PTSD) symptoms. It appeared that repeated discussions of prognosis in the ICU setting enhanced the experience of PTSD of family members.

Critical thinking involves paying attention to the relevant information involved. Excessive information makes it difficult to pay attention to what is important.

In an information-rich world, the wealth of information means a dearth of something else: a scarcity of whatever it is that information consumes. What information consumes is rather obvious: it consumes the attention of its recipients. Hence **a wealth of information creates a poverty of attention.**
—Herbert Simon (1916–1991), American political and computer scientist
(emphasis added)[1]

Reference

1. Simon H. Designing organizations for an information-rich world. In M Greenberger ed., *Computers, Communications, and the Public Interest*. Johns Hopkins University Press; 1971:38–73.

Lesson 20
Treat the Patient, Not the Test

It is critical to assess the significance of abnormal lab test results. The laboratory standards for normal values may not apply to your patient because of their age and other factors. For example, hemoglobin levels are inversely associated with age (healthy older persons have lower values than younger persons).[1]

Lab values are clues to what is going on with the patient. They must be considered in the full context of the patient's situation. Imagine a patient with epilepsy for many years who is doing well on medication but whose electroencephalogram (EEG) has some abnormal slow wave activity. Most neurologists would not advise a change in a successful medication regimen based on the EEG alone if the patient is doing well.

The need for frequent regular testing of anticoagulant plasma levels in patients who are doing well has also been questioned. Remember the danger of an "incidentaloma," a radiological abnormality found incidentally and of questionable significance. It may refer to an incidental mass in the adrenal gland, pituitary, thyroid, or other areas.[2] These findings may precipitate biopsies or other surgery which can have significant complications. Unnecessary distress and radiation exposure may result. Biopsy or surgery for these lesions should be carefully considered because of the risks involved.

Do not assume that all tests are accurate. It is important to be aware of the limitations of the testing. For example, an MRI scan of the brain in a 78-year-old person may show atrophy in the cortex. This may be found in persons with Alzheimer's disease. It is also commonly found in healthy older persons who are not cognitively impaired. It can be hazardous for the interpretation of the scan to be performed by a radiologist who has limited experience with patients.

Many older persons have knee and low back pain. MRI scans may document in detail degeneration in the intervertebral discs, foramina, and cartilage. (The foramina are openings between the vertebral bodies through which nerve roots travel.) What should be done with the patient cannot be determined independently through the MRI results. Well over 50% of all persons over 60 years of age have significant degeneration in the lumbar spine, as well as in the knees. Most people with back pain will get better with rest and physical therapy, without surgery. Of course, there are clinical and radiological findings which can indicate the urgent need for surgery, but, in all cases, imaging needs to be considered in the full context of the patient.

It is important to understand that biomarkers are signposts of disease, but are not disease itself (Lessons 20 and 45).

Test every concept by the question, "What sensible difference to anybody will its truth make?"

—William James[3]

References

1. Salive ME, Cornoni-Huntley J, Guralnik JM, Phillips CL, Wallace RB, Ostfeld AM, Cohen HJ. Anemia and hemoglobin levels in older persons: Relationship with age, gender, and health status. *J Am Geriatr Soc*. 1992 May;40(5):489–96. doi:10.1111/j.1532-5415.1992.tb02017.x. PMID: 1634703.
2. Reidelberger K, Fingeret A. Management of incidentalomas. *Surg Clin North Am*. 2021 Dec;101(6):1081–96. doi:10.1016/j.suc.2021.06.006. PMID: 34774270.
3. James W. *Some Problems of Philosophy*. Harvard University Press; 1911.

Lesson 21
It's Good To Be Knowledgeable, but It Is Necessary to Also Be Attentive to the Patient

Textbooks are poor representations of reality. In describing a disease, a textbook is not able to discuss all the various features of an illness with all their complexity and variability. If a photo shows a sign of an illness in a textbook or paper, it will most commonly be a relatively clear-cut and obvious illustration, often a severe case. A questionable or difficult-to-interpret image is not best for teaching. Although you must learn from reading textbooks, journals, and other media-based forms, you must realize that diagnosis and management of human disease is more complicated than can be perfectly described in writing. You need to learn from patients.

For example, consider pharmacology, which is a complex science. Physicians need to know about the chemical properties of the drugs they use, as well as the way the agents are handled by the body (*pharmacokinetics*) and what the drugs do to the body (*pharmacodynamics*). We need to consider how these processes are influenced by liver and kidney function, fluid balance, protein binding, competition with other drugs, and other issues. Of course, it is good to know about all these things. It is critical also to pay attention to how the patient is using the drugs. It is unfortunately often forgotten that drugs won't work if they are not taken in the correct manner. Evaluation of the patient's compliance with their medications is often overlooked and always necessary. Patients do not take their medications in the proper manner in more than 40% of cases (*noncompliance*, Lesson 14).[1]

An 82-year-old woman with hypertension is taking four drugs. A good clinician must consider the following for each: indications (were they good choices?), metabolism in the liver, excretion by the kidneys, binding in the plasma, potentials for interactions, possibility of addiction, cost, and other factors. All these factors may be important. However, the critical factor may be that the patient doesn't understand or doesn't remember how they should be taken. What time of day? With food or without food? And, if she does have a memory problem, she may not remember that she took them and take too much on some days and too little on other days. Attention focused on the patient is every bit as important as attention to the sciences of medicine.

The point of this lesson is that knowledge of anatomy, physiology, pharmacology, pathology, microbiology, genetics, and the like is all-important in patient care. But knowledge of the facts of these disciplines is not enough. It is necessary to know how your application of the sciences of medicine is influenced by the special features of the patient and the context of his life. This requires awareness of the patient and attention to his unique story.

> Do as much as possible for the patient, and as little as possible to the patient.
> —Bernard Lown, Founder, Lown Institute[2]

> He who studies medicine without books sails an uncharted sea, but he who studies medicine without patients does not go to sea at all.
> —William Osler

References

1. Osterberg L, Blaschke T. Adherence to medication. *N Engl J Med*. 2005 Aug 4;353(5):487-97. doi:10.1056/NEJMra050100. PMID: 16079372.
2. Lown Hospitals. About. Lown Institute Hospital Index. (n.d.). https://lownhospitalsindex.org/about/

Lesson 22
Consider Toxic Exposures

Toxic exposures may include heavy metals, solvents, pesticides, alcohol, and myriad other molecules. Many people underestimate their use of alcohol. Toxic exposures may be experienced at work, at home, or while involved in recreational activities. Women may suffer toxic exposures through the handling of their husbands' clothes. I had a female patient with a complex neurodegenerative disease with unusual features similar to Parkinson's disease leading to death at 72 years of age. There was no evidence of toxic exposures or family history of neurological illnesses. Her husband was a landscape designer. Two years after she died, I happened to visit another patient in her home and my former patient's husband came to work in my patient's garden. I was shocked to see that he used large amounts of herbicides and pesticides without any protective equipment whatsoever and that he had these chemicals loosely stored in vats in the trunk of his car. When he sprayed the garden he seemed to have no awareness that he was spraying his pants and shoes at the same time. It's possible that her illness was caused or exacerbated by exposures to his clothing and to his car with its toxic environment. It might be argued that occupational exposure such as this would affect the husband before it would affect his wife because his exposure was more intense. This reasoning is erroneous because it neglects the contribution of genetics and epigenetics.[1] (*Epigenetics* is the study of the modifications of genes that do not alter the genetic code.)

If there is a possible toxic exposure at work, it may be necessary to write to the workplace asking for information about the patient's possible exposures. Permission from the patient is required before such a request can be made. Evaluation of possible exposures requires detailed questioning. A patient who is an accountant may sit at a desk in an office with no potential danger of toxic exposures. An accountant may also have an office in a factory and be in contact with fumes and other pollutants. The role of exposures can be difficult to evaluate as many persons may have suffered exposures decades ago, when occupational protections were less effective.

Pottery made using lead-containing glaze can cause exposure upon repeated use. Supplements and herbal preparations may also contain toxins. To evaluate the possibility of toxic exposures it is necessary to get to know the patient and the patient's lifestyle (Lesson 57).

I had a patient with features of both Alzheimer's disease and motor neuron disease who worked in a foundry pouring molten aluminum.[1] To document the effect of the heavy metal exposure on his disease a brain biopsy was done by a neurosurgeon using

---

[1] It is known that aluminum injected into the brain is highly toxic.

a plastic knife so that metal from the surgical instrument would not influence the assessment of metal content in the brain. To my surprise the assay showed that aluminum and other metals were not present in the tissue. Aluminum is the third most abundant metal in the earth's crust, and we evolved with this potentially dangerous exposure. This required us to develop excellent protective mechanisms against entry of aluminum into the body and the brain.

It is often assumed that toxic exposures will affect the nervous system diffusely and symmetrically. This may often be the case but is not always correct. In Lesson 93, the effect of 1-methyl-4-phenyl-1,2,3,6-tetrahydropyridine (MPTP) exposure on specific degeneration of motor neurons in the substantia nigra is discussed. Toxic exposures can also have focal effects because of their interaction with pre-existing deficits in reserve capacity.

The good physician treats the disease: the great physician treats the patient who has the disease.

—Attributed to William Osler

Reference

1. Collotta M, Bertazzi PA, Bollati V. Epigenetics and pesticides. *Toxicology*. 2013 May 10;307:35–41. doi:10.1016/j.tox.2013.01.017. Epub 2013 Feb 1. PMID: 23380243.

Lesson 23
Family History Is an Important Part of the Interview

In medicine, we are generally concerned with family history involving first-degree relatives (parents, children, brothers, and sisters). It is common that family members may have inherited conditions with limited awareness of the meaning of their family's history. For example, a patient of mine with familial amyotrophic lateral sclerosis had one ancestor who was said to have had "creeping paralysis" and another who was misdiagnosed as having Parkinson's disease.

It is best to get the family history from as many members of the family as possible. Also, family history should be obtained on more than one visit. It is advisable to ask the patient and family members to describe the medical history of the patient's father, mother, siblings, and children. This is more thorough than only asking if there are any inherited disorders in the family.

A patient was being seen with a new diagnosis of Charcot-Marie-Tooth disease. This is a progressive disease of the peripheral nerves, named after the doctors who first reported it in 1886 (Jean Marie Charcot, Pierre Marie, and Howard Tooth). It is associated with weakness in the legs and hands and skinny legs. The patient was asked if anyone in her family had any neurological condition, and she said no. The neurologist asked the patient's uncle, who was with her, if he would please raise the legs of his pants, so his shins could be examined. It was shown that he also had the characteristic atrophy found with the disease, referred to as "stork legs" (*atrophy* is loss of muscle bulk). This important aspect of the family history would not have been available if the uncle had not attended the visit.

A patient without a family history of neurological disease may still have a genetic condition. The genetic change may be a new mutation, or there may be false paternity (the patient's father is not one the one believed to be the father). The rate of false paternity may be as high as 2–5%. (The occurrence of false maternity is much lower!) It is a mistake to assume that a condition does not have genetic features because of the patient's advanced age. I saw a patient with mild chorea beginning at 72 years of age caused by Huntington's disease (*chorea* is an involuntary movement of the arms or legs which is sudden and jerky).

> To forget one's ancestors is to be a brook without a source, a tree without a root.
> —Chinese Proverb

Lesson 24
Rare Presentations of Common Events Are More Common Than Common Presentations of Rare Events

A 56-year-old woman came to see me with memory loss and prominent visual problems. She could no longer drive a car, was walking into things, and falling because of tripping on objects she did not notice. She saw an ophthalmologist who could find nothing wrong with her eyes. The problems had been progressive over the previous 10 months. MRI scan of the brain showed atrophy of the cortex in the posterior occipital and parietal lobes. The differential diagnosis included the posterior cortical variant of Alzheimer's disease, in which visual problems are prominent because of the involvement of the visual processing areas of the occipital lobes. Creutzfeldt-Jakob disease, associated with occipital lesions and visual dysfunction, was another consideration.

Clinical judgment demands that we evaluate the probability of potential explanations. We should not assume that something cannot happen because it is uncommon. An important consideration is that common problems occur frequently, of course, so that unusual presentations of common things are more common than the usual presentation of a rare condition. Creutzfeldt-Jakob disease prevalence is approximately 1 per million. Alzheimer's disease is also a cause of dementia and is much more common, affecting more than 3% of people worldwide over the age of 65.[1] This means that for every million people 65 years of age and older there will be more than 30,000 people with Alzheimer's disease and only one person with Creutzfeldt-Jakob disease. So, if only 1% of people with Alzheimer's disease has a certain unusual phenotype (observable traits) such as mode of presentation, speed of progression, or distribution of cognitive deficits, there will be a thousand people with those characteristics. This led us to consider that our patient with dementia with visual dysfunction most likely had the posterior cortical atrophy variant of Alzheimer's disease. Of course, neuroimaging and cerebrospinal fluid (CSF) tests were also needed to confirm the diagnosis.

Reference

1. Alzheimer's Disease International. Alzheimer's disease international dementia statistics. https://www.alzint.org/about/dementia-facts-figures/dementia-statistics/. Accessed Nov 2, 2023.

Lesson 25
Symptoms and Signs Have Important Significance

The Absence of Symptoms and Signs Is Not Always as Important as Their Presence

In the study of medicine, we learn about the symptoms and signs of pneumonia: fever, cough, difficulty breathing, abnormal breath sounds, chest pain, increased white blood cell count, and chest X-ray changes, among other signs. The presence of these symptoms, signs, and laboratory abnormalities suggests that pneumonia may be present. The absence of these signs does not have equivalent significance indicating that pneumonia is not present. It is most correct to say that the absence of fever, abnormal breath sounds, and chest X-ray abnormalities suggests that pneumonia is not present. However, it does not exclude the possibility that the patient has pneumonia. If a test suggests that a disorder is not present when it is present, it is called a *false-negative test*.

The presence of a Babinski sign suggests that there is a contralateral lesion in the upper motor neuron (the pyramidal tract). The absence of a Babinski sign does not mean that there is no lesion in this motor system.

A paper in the *New England Journal of Medicine* reported a 44-year-old man who went to the emergency room with severe pain after dropping a 200-kilogram bar in the gym on his lower back.[1] He could crawl out from under the weight but could not walk. He had full power in both legs and normal sensation in all dermatomes in his legs. The area over vertebral bodies T11 through L2 was tender, and an X-ray showed a fracture dislocation of the spine from the lower thoracic to upper lumbar region. (Dislocation means that the spinal canal was significantly misaligned.) Surgery was done with good preservation of neurological function. The fact that he retained motion and sensation in his legs suggested that he did not have a fracture dislocation of the spine. But for some reason his spinal cord retained function even though the spinal canal through which it passed was severely disrupted.

Splinter hemorrhages under the fingernails is a sign of endocarditis. The lack of splinter hemorrhages does not mean that a patient does not have endocarditis. Patients with intracranial bleeding will most often have evidence of red blood cells in the cerebrospinal fluid (CSF). The absence of blood in the CSF does not mean that a patient did not have an intracranial hemorrhage. Pain in the right lower part of the abdomen is a sign of appendicitis. The absence of abdominal pain does not mean that a person cannot be suffering with appendicitis (appendicitis can also cause low back pain!).

I have seen four cases of dementia where the patients had brain tumors without focal abnormality of movement, sensation, or papilledema (swelling of the optic nerve head suggestive of increased intracranial pressure). Because the tumors were slow-growing it was possible for the brain to adapt to their presence for many years without symptoms. When this adaptation was no longer possible, dementia developed.

An alcoholic patient came to the emergency room after falling down the stairs. He had neck pain and remarkable rigidity of his neck, with no problem with motor or sensory function in his arms or legs. An urgent X-ray of his cervical spine showed a non-displaced fracture of the lower cervical spine. His rigidity was an involuntary response to stabilize the spine. The fact that he had no signs in his legs of weakness or sensory loss did not mean that his spine was not fractured.

Reference

1. Evans LJ. Images in clinical medicine: Thoracolumbar fracture with preservation of neurologic function. *N Engl J Med.* 2012 Nov 15;367(20):1939. doi:10.1056/NEJMicm1101495. PMID: 23150961.

Lesson 26
Salutogenesis
The Production and Maintenance of Health

The concept of *salutogenesis*, the production and maintenance of health, contrasts with the concept of *pathogenesis*, which is the initiation and maintenance of disease. "*Salutogenesis*—of the origins (*genesis*) of health (*saluto*)."[1]. The salutogenesis concept was developed by Aaron Antonovsky (1923–1994), an Israeli American sociologist who agreed with Victor Frankl that a sense of meaning was an important part of health.

Health is not only the absence of disease. It's possible to have two patients who are both equally free of disease, with one being considerably healthier than the other. (One may be significantly overweight, with poor physical fitness, poor pulmonary capacity, and poorer cognitive reserve capacity.) Fitness is an important component of health that determines our *resilience* (reserve capacity), which is the ability to stay healthy despite negative forces that we experience with aging. I have proposed four aspects of this resilience called the *multiple reserves*: cognitive, physical, psychological, and social. The maintenance and enhancement of these four reserves is a key aspect of healthy aging, as I discuss in my book, *Unaging: The Four Factors That Impact How You Age*.[2]

It would be much more effective if the healthcare professions were dedicated to keeping people healthy rather than only taking care of them when they are ill.

Consider herpes zoster, also called shingles. It is a viral infection in the dorsal root ganglia which causes considerable pain and disability. A vaccine is available in the United States for persons 50 years of age or older and it is highly effective in reducing the risk of developing the infection. I advise all of my patients of that age group to have the vaccine because I believe that I should do whatever I can to help them maintain their health. Other aspects of neurological prevention which I discuss with my patients include a low saturated fat, high-fiber diet, avoidance of head injury, good levels of oral care, high levels of physical activity and cognitive stimulation at home and at work, and good control of hypertension.[2]

It is my experience that neurologists do not commonly recommend the zoster vaccine, perhaps because patients do not come in with the chief complaint of "Doctor can you please tell me how I can avoid getting herpes zoster?" It is also clear that poor oral health is a risk factor for heart disease, stroke, and Alzheimer's disease, as well as other conditions. It takes little time and no expense for a physician to explain the importance of taking care of their teeth to all patients. My experience is that oral health is rarely mentioned in clinic visits (except for appointments with the dentist).

Neurologists and many specialists are not often concerned with prevention. To think critically about health care, we need to go beyond disease management and consider the salutogenic approach: how can persons be helped at each stage of life to achieve and maintain health and enhance meaning?

—Aaron Antonovsky[3]

References

1. Mittelmark MB, Sagy S, Eriksson M, Bauer GF, Pelikan JM, Lindström B, Espnes GA, eds. *The Handbook of Salutogenesis*. Springer; 2017. PMID: 28590610.
2. Friedland RP *Unaging: The Four Factors That Impact How You Age*. University of Cambridge Press; 2022.
3. Vinje HF, Langeland E, Bull T. Aaron Antonovsky's development of salutogenesis, 1979 to 1994. In Mittelmark MB, Sagy S, Eriksson M, et al., eds. *The Handbook of Salutogenesis*. Springer; 2017: chapter 4. https://www.ncbi.nlm.nih.gov/books/NBK435860/ doi:10.1007/978-3-319-04600-6_4

SECTION III
MANAGEMENT

Lesson 27
Get to Know the Patient and Show Interest (the Patient Is a Person)

Getting to know the patient shows that you are concerned about their care. Furthermore, the more you know about the patient the more you can provide them with comprehensive, compassionate care. It is vital to obtain a full social history in each case so that you know the patient's education level, occupational attainment, and recreational activities (as well as their level of alcohol intake and other toxic exposures). Obtaining information about the patient's life will help you assess possible environmental factors that influence disease. Having them talk about their own interests will help to establish a healthy relationship. I had a patient who was a fabric artist, and, at every visit, I would discuss her current work. Another patient was a trainer of thoroughbred horses, and I would ask him how his horses were doing. We must show the patient that we consider them more than a composite of organs.

Getting to know the patient may also provide a clue to possible toxic exposures and help you evaluate their cognitive capacity. Knowing about their ability to understand complex concepts will help you give them instructions about medication use and lifestyle factors.

It is not possible to take care of the patient properly if you don't learn about them.[1] Features of genetic background, education, recreational activities, injuries, toxic exposures, trauma, and upbringing can all be important and worthy of consideration. You may have the right diagnosis and the right treatment, but if you're giving it to the wrong patient, it won't be effective.

It is valuable to take time to get to know who the patient is. I was seeing a 72-year-old man with dementia for the first time. He was not happy to be in my clinic because his family hadn't told him that he was coming to see a doctor specializing in memory deficits. He thought that there was nothing wrong with his cognitive capacity. It is common, of course, that many persons with dementia do not know they have a memory problem, perhaps because they forget that they are forgetting. He was agitated and got up to leave when I came in the room, I said hello and he responded with obscenities telling me that there was nothing *blank-blank-blank* wrong with him. I noticed a tattoo on his arm; I held his hand to see it better and asked him where he got it. He told me that he got drunk in Belgium during World War II in the army and woke up in the morning with this tattoo. I asked him questions about his war experience. After several minutes of this interaction, he forgot that he hated me. He also forgot that he didn't want to be there. He had shared a very important aspect of his life history and that helped to improve our relationship.

I often need to consider whether a patient with a stroke or dementia with a communication problem will benefit from referral to speech or physical therapy. I nearly always recommend such therapy because there is evidence supporting its use. There are mechanisms of brain plasticity involving repair, rebuilding, and establishment of brain networks that are enhanced by activities involved in therapy. *Plasticity* refers to the ability of being soft enough to be changed into a new shape. In neuroscience, it describes the ability of neurons and their networks to be improved through experience.

I saw a powerful example of the value of physical therapy involving an 80-year-old man with left hemiparesis (weakness on the left side of the body). His physical therapist came to see him in the hospital and asked him to elevate his shoulder. He did so to a minimal degree. The therapist complimented him in a loud voice saying that the improvement was excellent. The therapist called out to another physical therapist telling her to come look what he can do—"Isn't that great?" Depression is a common complication of stroke. Certainly, a powerful emotional and physical connection with the therapist can help improve the patient's mood, enhance participation in therapy, and enhance recovery.

Speech and physical therapy are almost always helpful. The brain is remarkably adaptable and reorganizes in response to injury. The psychological effect of having a caring person interested in the patient is of great value.

> In my view, the lost art of listening and ignoring the patient as a human being is a quintessential failure of our health care.
>
> —Bernard Lown[1]

> What is the meaning of a human being? In dealing with a particular man I do not come upon a generality but upon an individuality, upon uniqueness, upon a person. I see a face, not only a body; a special situation, not a typical case. The disease is common, the patient is unique.
>
> —Rabbi Abraham Joshua Heschel[2]

> It is more important to know what kind of patient has the disease than it is to know what kind of disease the patient has.
>
> —Attributed to Hippocrates

References

1. Lown B. *The Lost Art of Healing: Practicing Compassion in Medicine*. Ballantine Books; 1999.
2. Heschel AJ. The patient as a person. In *The Insecurity of Freedom: Essays on Human Existence*. Noonday; 1967:24–38.
3. Centor RM. To be a great physician, you must understand the whole story. *MedGenMed*. 2007 Mar 26;9(1):59. PMID: 17435659; PMCID: PMC1924990.

Lesson 28
Learn from Clinical Experience (but Not Too Much)

Clinical experience is what you learn from your patients over the course of your career. It is enormously important, of course, in making you a good doctor. The quality of your clinical experience depends on the ferocity of your attention to your patients and their disease course and outcomes. If you only see patients once, your clinical experience will be limited by a lack of information about what happened to them. If you do not make efforts to find out what transpires with your patients, your clinical experience database will be impaired. Your job is to respect the value of your clinical experience and see that you enhance it consistently. Your clinical experience helps to make you a better doctor only if you devote yourself to paying attention to your patients.

It is critical to recognize that clinical experience is always incomplete. Individual physicians do not see a random representation of the public. There are always factors such as geography, finances, ethnicity, insurance, language, specialization, and other matters which influence who shows up in your office as well as who returns. Also, you must realize that your clinical experience is limited by the number of patients you see. That is, if you treat three patients with a new drug and they all do poorly, it could be that the drug is a poor choice for their condition. Or it may be an excellent choice for their condition but not for these particular patients, who were misdiagnosed, or at the wrong stage of their illness, or had comorbidity (other illnesses). Perhaps this new treatment is effective in 80% of cases with this condition, but the three patients you treated happened to be in the 20% who do not respond.

This matter does not mean that clinical experience is ignored, but instead that these limitations must always be considered.

Lesson 29
Use the Placebo Response to Your Patient's Benefit

If you have reason to believe that a therapy will work, you should explain this to the patient in a positive way. You need to discuss side effects, but you should not exaggerate the risks. If you read the exhaustive information available in the prescribing information to each patient, nobody would ever agree to take any drug. Although you must be honest concerning risks, you should be aware that patients may do better if they have positive expectations. At least one-third of all drug effects are produced by placebo effects. Placebo effects also can apply to surgery as well as physical therapy and rehabilitation.[1] Furthermore, a negative effect (the *nocebo effect*) is possible when there is a negative response to an agent caused by the expectation that it will not do well. It is important that both patient and family have an accurate expectation of the effects of drugs and surgery.

Reference

1. Probst P, Grummich K, Harnoss JC, Hüttner FJ, Jensen K, Braun S, Kieser M, Ulrich A, Büchler MW, Diener MK. Placebo-controlled trials in surgery: A systematic review and meta-analysis. *Medicine*. 2016;95(17):e3516. https://doi.org/10.1097/MD.0000000000003516

Lesson 30
Tell the Truth Whenever Possible

Be honest, so that the patient can trust you. If you believe that the patient will be harmed by giving them truthful information, you are rarely allowed to misrepresent the true situation. If your patient has vertigo and ear pain, you may choose to order an MRI of the brain. If the patient asks you why, you can say that you wish to examine the structure of the inner ear. You do not need to tell them that you are checking for the possibility that they have a brain tumor (acoustic neuroma), although this is a possible outcome. If the patient is in the emergency room with chest pain and the EKG shows unusually high ST segment elevation suggestive of an acute myocardial infarction (heart attack), you do not need to tell the patient about the severity of the finding. You might tell them that it does show a problem which is going to be treated in the ICU. A bioethicist discusses his decision to lie to his 87-year-old mother with apparent cancer in the short essay "Lying to my mom," in the *Journal of the American Medical Association*.[1]

It is generally best to be honest when telling patients their diagnosis. Support from the family and from friends is critical. It is wise to assess the patient's ability to understand. However, even with Alzheimer's, most patients should be told of their diagnosis. It is helpful for them to replace the uncertainty of not knowing what's wrong with them with having a name to account for their difficulties. It is uncommon for dementia patients to have a bad reaction to being told of their diagnosis. There are occasions when the patient's understanding is poor and being told that they have Alzheimer's may not be advisable. As dementia progresses in Alzheimer's disease it may be desirable to mislead the patient. A nursing home in the Netherlands observed that many patients were "sundowning" in the afternoon and consistently insisting on going home. (*Sundowning* is a state of confusion in the late afternoon experienced by patients with dementia.) The care workers had a realistic bus stop installed next to the home, and they would gather those patients who wish to go home to go outside to catch the bus. The bus was actually not ever coming. They would wait about 30 minutes and then say "I guess the bus is not coming today, let's go inside and have a cup of tea." The patients would be generally agreeable to this outcome because they had forgotten their expectation of going home.[2]

In deciding what to tell the patient about serious conditions, realize that the spouse is not the patient. Your primary obligation is to the patient. You must, of course, discuss the situation with the next of kin, but you are not required to always follow the wishes of the companion.

It is advisable to give honest answers to the patient's questions. A trusting relationship between the patient and medical professional is critical.

References

1. Feudtner C. Lying to my mom. *JAMA*. 2023 Oct 10;330(14):1333–4. doi:10.1001/jama.2023.17581. PMID: 37728956.
2. Lorey P. Fake bus stops for persons with dementia? On truth and benevolent lies in public health. *Isr J Health Policy Res*. 2019 Mar 7;8(1):28. doi:10.1186/s13584-019-0301-0. PMID: 30845988; PMCID: PMC6407192.

Lesson 31
Cognitive Function Is Relevant for All Areas of Medicine

Assessment of mental function is an important part of neurology, psychiatry, psychology, and neurosurgery. However, a urologist needs to know about the patient's mental cognitive abilities if she is going to give the patient a choice of therapies for prostate cancer. For example, will the patient prefer freezing, heating, open surgery, robotic surgery, radiotherapy beads, or conventional radiotherapy? If the patient is not capable of understanding these complex concepts, he should not be the one making the decision.

Every patient who signs a consent form in the hospital, including the consent for admission, is required to be competent to be eligible to give consent. If you're instructing a patient on how to self-administer insulin based on blood sugar recordings, you need to know that they're able to understand your instructions to carry them out. All physicians need to know how to evaluate the patient's competence to make decisions. Competence involves memory as well as understanding. To be able to make decisions for their own care the patient must have sufficient memory and comprehension so that they can properly understand their condition and the prospects for the planned interventions.

Lesson 32
You Are Primarily Responsible for Caring for the Patient, Not the Family

The physician is responsible for the care of the patient. This includes learning about the family and other caregivers. Although the interests and wishes of the patient's family need to be considered, it is important to recognize that the patient's care is the primary factor, not the concerns of the family. Most of the time it is certainly true that the family has the best interest of the patient in mind. However, this is not always the case. There may be situations in which family members would like to have access to the patients' financial resources. Because of this they may desire to have the patient inappropriately declared incompetent. And it may rarely happen that family members seek the demise of the patient through withholding of care or delivery of inappropriate care.

It is a particularly difficult situation when members of the family do not agree. Assistance in such cases from social workers, hospital administrators, and attorneys may be advisable. The critical matter is to be aware of the possibility that the family may not have the best interest of the patient in mind.

A most tragic example of this issue is the death of neurologist Dr. Autumn Klein, who was poisoned by her husband with cyanide at the age of 41. Her husband was a neuroscience researcher at the University of Pittsburgh who is serving a life sentence for first-degree murder.[1]

Reference

1. Ward PR. *Death by Cyanide: The Murder of Dr. Autumn Klein P. Ward*. ForeEdge; 2016.

Lesson 33
Denial of Illness and Disability Can Be Shared by the Patient, the Family, and the Doctor

No one likes to be sick; family members don't want loved ones to be sick, and the doctor doesn't want the patient to be sick. Denial can also affect the community. US President Ronald Reagan was diagnosed with Alzheimer's disease after leaving office (in 1994). It is clear that he suffered from significant memory disturbances in both of his two terms of office. The implications of his cognitive impairment were denied by him, his family, his doctors, and the nation.[1]

Denial can be explicit or implicit. Explicit denial occurs when the patient is not able to acknowledge any awareness of the deficit. In *implicit denial*, there is a lack of recognition of the full nature and importance of the deficit at the same time that the patient shows awareness to some degree. The patient with explicit denial will say there is nothing wrong with them. A patient with implicit denial may acknowledge a problem but say that its cause is trivial and not significant. Recognition of both forms of denial is critical for planning therapy and monitoring progress.

Denial of illness can affect any aspect of human health. Although the literature concerning denial of illness has focused on neurological disorders,[2] it is also highly relevant to other of the body's systems. Patients who are significantly obese may feel it is not a problem because they have lost weight. Hypertensive patients may fail to recognize the importance of blood pressure monitoring, and diabetics may eat badly and improperly administer their medications. Persons with skin cancers may fail to seek help until the lesions start bleeding. I had a patient with breast cancer who did not come in to see a doctor until the tumor had eroded through the skin. Similarly, smokers might believe they do not have a problem with smoking because they have cut back from three to one pack a day (all levels of smoking exposure are hazardous).

Denial of illness is a very basic defense mechanism which plays a pivotal role in human health.[2] The presence of denial can result in incorrect information about the patient's condition and abilities. Denial can also interfere with use of medications and compliance with suggested actions. It is essential to be aware of the reality that the patient and family may not recognize the serious nature of what is happening. **If it were possible to determine the magnitude of the impact of denial, we would be surprised to see that denial is a major cause of death.**

Providers of medical care must assess the degree to which the patient and family understand the significance of their symptoms, signs, diagnosis, and treatment plan. Both implicit and explicit denial can interfere with the patient's compliance with care monitoring and therapy.

References

1. Reagan R Jr. *My Father at 100: A Memoir*. Viking; 2011.
2. Weinstein EA, Kahn RL. *Denial of Illness: Symbolic and Physiological Aspects*. Charles C. Thomas, 1955. https://doi.org/10.1037/11516-000

Lesson 34
Consider the Context of Care

> All three levels, biological, psychological and social must be taken into account in every health care task.
>
> —G. L. Engel[1]

The word "context" comes from a Latin phrase "to weave together" (to fabricate) (Online Etymology Dictionary). Consideration of context in healthcare and in scientific endeavors is critical. When decisions are made, we need to evaluate biological, psychological, and social factors which may be important. Contextualizing care involves focusing on communication and thinking skills. What questions do we ask, and do we listen carefully to the answers? Do we consider the patient's life circumstances and how they influence care?[2]

The context of care considers individual differences. If you tell a 70-year-old alcoholic patient that he needs to stop drinking alcohol, you need to know if his wife is also alcoholic. (It is difficult for a person to stop drinking alcohol if they live with someone who is drinking excessively.) It may not help to tell a patient who is chronically late for appointments that she must come to clinic on time without knowing that she drives 3 hours to every appointment and that her appointments have all been early in the morning.

The issue of context is also relevant to scientific investigations. Clearly, Galileo had to consider the reaction of the Church to his great discoveries. Hungarian physician Ignaz Semmelweis failed to consider the hostile reaction of the medical establishment to his insistence that doctors and nurses all wash their hands between patients. How could a proposal for hand-washing be rejected? Let us consider what happened in Vienna around 1850–1865.

Ignaz Semmelweis was a Hungarian physician who observed that the rate of death from childbed fever (also called *puerperal fever*) was much higher in women who gave birth in the hospital with the assistance of doctors compared to women who gave birth at home or with the help of midwives.[3,*] In the 1850s, the death rate in the Vienna hospital where Semmelweis worked was so high that women would try to give birth in the street before being brought to the hospital. Semmelweis proposed that hand-washing would prevent disease transmission. He was aware of Louis Pasteur's work on the germ theory of disease, and he also learned from observing the death of a colleague from sepsis after he had cut himself in the autopsy room.[†] At the time

---

[*] It is now known that most cases of puerperal fever are caused by infection with *Streptococci*.
[†] Sepsis is a life-threatening condition when infection spreads in the circulation.

doctors would go from the delivery room to the morgue and then back to the delivery room without washing their hands. Their white coats were often covered in blood and were not frequently changed because the magnitude of the stains on their coats was a sign of the success of their medical practice. The new mandatory hand-washing practices lowered the mortality rate by more than 90%. Despite this positive outcome his focus on cleanliness was met with stiff resistance from the medical establishment, and he was dismissed from his hospital position and forced to leave Vienna and move to Budapest. At the time it was believed that childbed fever was caused by "uncleanliness of the bowel" and bad air (miasma). Semmelweis's work was even rejected by Rudolf Virchow, a leading physician of the time (Lesson 4).

The bacterial mechanisms responsible for childbed fever were only uncovered after Semmelweis's death, when the new germ theory of disease developed by Louis Pasteur and Joseph Lister was established (1860s–1870s). Contributing to Semmelweis's problems were his slow speed of publication and his angry and aggressive assaults on his colleagues. Acceptance of his important work would have been enhanced if he had considered the context of his proposals. The reflex-like rejection of new knowledge because it contradicts existing belief has been called the *Semmelweis reflex*.

D. L. Rosenhan (1929–2012) was a Stanford University psychologist who did an experiment challenging the truth of psychiatric diagnoses. In a 1973 *Science* paper "On being sane in insane places,"[4] he had nine research participants go to psychiatric hospitals pretending to hear voices in their heads in order to get admitted. Other than the voices, they talked about true events in their own lives. When they were admitted they stopped reporting voices and did nothing that would be considered abnormal. The pseudopatients were instructed to "act normally." Most were diagnosed as schizophrenic and one as manic depressive. The treating psychiatrist did not recognize that the so-called patients were not insane and treated them with antipsychotic medications. Remarkably, many of the other patients correctly identified them as impostors. Importantly, the pseudopatients reported experiencing dehumanization, with invasions of privacy and boredom. Patient matters were discussed in their presence as though they were not there, and they experienced verbal and physical abuse. Rosenhan wished hospitals to be more aware of the social psychology of their facilities. The context of the patient's presentation to the hospital was the key factor in their misdiagnosis.

A disturbing example of the role of context in healthcare is consideration of the relationship between social economic status and risk of dementing illness. All lifestyle factors that increase risk for Alzheimer's disease and related dementing disorders are more common in disadvantaged neighborhoods: diets high in saturated fat and salt, lower levels of physical activity, lower levels of education, toxic exposures at home and work (including air pollution), head injuries, poor dental hygiene, obesity, diabetes, hypertension, and, of course, impaired access to healthcare. These factors that contribute to the higher risk of Alzheimer's and related disorders in historically underrepresented and socially disadvantaged populations have been called the "social exposome."[5]

In a *Journal of the American Medical Association* article entitled "Dementia risk and disadvantaged neighborhoods," Dintica et al. conclude that "The social exposome should be addressed when interventions are developed because it is an essential factor associated with health disparities, reflecting systemic inequities within any society."[5] These factors are important for both public health and the care of individuals. We need to consider the social exposome to place the care of individual patients in the proper context.

The key to avoiding context errors is listening and asking the right questions. In *Listening for What Matters: Avoiding Contextual Errors in Health Care*, by S. J. Weiner and A. Schwarz, a patient's context is defined "as everything expressed outside the skin that is relevant to planning their care."[2] This all-encompassing concept includes practical considerations and all the social and cultural dimensions of a person's life that impact their role as a patient and their interaction with caregivers.

Ignac Semmelweis (1818–1865): A Person to Know

Semmelweis was a Hungarian physiologist and scientist and an early developer of antiseptic procedures (preventing the growth of disease-causing microorganisms).[3] His studies, which were highly controversial at the time, illustrated the importance of cleanliness and the danger of transmission of infectious material from patient to patient or from the morgue to the clinic. His work was not initially accepted in either Vienna or Budapest, and he was rejected for an assistant professor position in Vienna and returned to Budapest. He was put in a mental hospital, where he died from sepsis in 1865. His final illness may have been caused by a beating from the guards. After his death Louis Pasteur and Joseph Lister confirmed his ideas and provided convincing evidence of the importance of antisepsis.[6]

> Should you, Herr Hofrath, without having disproved my doctrine, continue to train your pupils [against it], I declare before God and the world that you are a murderer and the "History of Childbed Fever" would not be unjust to you if it memorialized you as a medical Nero.
> —Letter of Semmelweis to Dr. Eduard Hofrath, Vienna Professor of Surgery and opponent of Semmelweis's policy of antisepsis[7]

References

1. Ghaemi SN. *The Rise and Fall of the Biopsychosocial Model*. Johns Hopkins University Press; 2010.
2. SJ Weiner, Schwarz A. *Listening for What Matters: Avoiding Contextual Errors in Health Care*. Oxford University Press; 2016.

3. Nuland S. *The Doctors' Plague: Germs, Childbed Fever, and the Strange Story of Ignac Semmelweis*. Norton; 2003.
4. Rosenhan DL. On being sane in insane places. *Science*. 1973;179:250–8.
5. Dintica CS, Bahorik A, Xia F, Kind A, Yaffe K. Dementia risk and disadvantaged neighborhoods. *JAMA Neurol*. 2023 Sep 1;80(9):903–9. doi:10.1001/jamaneurol.2023.2120. Erratum in: JAMA Neurol. 2023 Sep 1;80(9):1004. PMID: 37464954; PMCID: PMC10357362.
6. Fitzharris L. *The Butchering Art: Joseph Lister's Quest to Transform the Grisly World of Victorian Medicine*. Farrar, Straus and Giroux; 2017.
7. Bhattacharya K. Ignaz Semmelweis: Handwashing invention and COVID-19. *Indian J Surg*. 2020 Jun;82(3):291–2. doi:10.1007/s12262-020-02445-y. Epub 2020 Jun 6. PMID: 32837066; PMCID: PMC7274934.

Lesson 35
Challenges to the Ability to Provide Humane Healthcare

Critical thinking describes our ability to gather information and make decisions guiding our actions and beliefs. Current developments in information systems are influencing all aspects of critical thinking processes. There is a danger that these changes are damaging the ability of physicians to provide person-centered care.

The electronic health record should be designed to help practitioners make good decisions and monitor the patient's progress. However, at the moment, the records are designed to enhance billing and not to enhance care.[1]

The record contains an enormous amount of extraneous information which is often redundant and has little or no relevance to clinical matters (Lesson 19). This problem was pointed out by Rabbi Abraham Joshua Heschel in a remarkable 1964 address to the American Medical Association. He said "Technology is growing apace ... soon the doctor may be obsolete. The data about the patient would be collected by camera and Dictaphone, or arranged by typists, processed into a computer."[2]

These developments foreseen by Rabbi Heschel are now well-established, and his fear that the doctor may become obsolete is well-founded. Shortly we will also have cameras in each exam room connected to a computer which will use artificial intelligence (AI) to analyze the verbal and visual aspects of the visit. It will likely be possible for an AI system to analyze the patient's tremor (for example) and say that the tremor is or is not suggestive of Parkinson's disease. The medical history may be completed by the computer's questioning of the patient. Will the primary role of the physician be preserved in this new system? I am skeptical.

It is critical that computer systems as well as AI programs evaluate the influence of the program on the doctor's cognitive load[3] (Lesson 19). The electronic health system should allow for rapid scanning of results. A complete blood count report should have abnormal values indicated in red so they can be quickly identified without having to read every value. If you get a result of your test back, the system should allow you to see the result without having to laboriously go to several locations in the record to obtain the report. The medications the patient takes should be listed in a clear manner. You do not need to know who ordered the medication or how many refills there are for every item. This information can be made available if requested. Ideally, you should be able to click on the name of the drug, and an explanation should then be provided. It should not be necessary to go to another information source to learn about a new drug that you have not previously encountered.

AI describes a scenario in which computers perform tasks that are usually done by humans.[4] The potential for AI systems to assist in healthcare is enormous, although its value in medical and scientific applications is just beginning to be explored. The growth of AI has been limited by the speed of available computing systems. This has become less of a problem with great advances in computing speed. It is now possible for a computer to mimic aspects of doctor–patient interactions.[4] Computer applications using machine learning methods to imitate the ways that humans learn have improved accuracy. This has been shown to be helpful for X-ray interpretation and analysis of retinal images and skin lesions, as well as electrocardiograms and MRI and positron emission tomography (PET) scans.[5]

AI systems are being explored for optimization of dementia diagnosis, prevention, and management. "Deep learning" systems have been shown to be of value in diagnosing Alzheimer's disease using information about gut bacteria.[5,*] There is a danger that the results of AI data analysis from patients with dementia will be misinterpreted by clinicians who are not experienced in the area.

It should be recognized that the performance levels of AI systems do not need to be as good as the most experienced and accomplished physicians, although that is desirable. Performance at a level better than most physicians will be helpful.

The use of advanced computer systems with support from humans taking responsibility for the training data is called *collaborative intelligence*.[3] Computer programs can use natural language processing to analyze questions and provide automated responses resembling a human conversation (such as ChatGTP from OpenAI).[4] The availability of enormous amounts of information on the internet can help the "chat box" to be extraordinarily informative. However, the results can be erroneous. When I looked myself up on ChatGPT I learned that, to my surprise, I was someone else. It will be necessary for the user of the chat box to analyze the accuracy of the report, which may be difficult to resolve.[5]

Several forms of bias can be found in AI programs. Generative AI models may contain established racial, gender, and class biases, which are strong factors involved in the fabrication of information. Biases in AI systems have been linked to *anchoring*, in which existing data dominate future analyses. (Lesson 51). AI systems may present existing biases concerning marginalized populations who will be affected by negative bias in outcomes.[6] Outputs need to be evaluated in consideration of this pervasive bias.[4] If the datasets are not representative of diversity, the applicability will be damaged.[7]

It has been recognized that AI systems have a problem distinguishing fact from fiction. These considerations are discussed in a 2023 *Science* paper "How AI can distort human beliefs: Models can convey biases and false information to users."[6]

It is important for physicians to understand the capacity of AI systems to be wrong. Clearly, it is vital that the results of AI analyses be carefully reviewed using human

---

* *Deep learning* is a variety of AI in which computers process data in a manner similar to that of the human brain. It is a version of machine learning using artificial neural networks to improve projections.

judgment. However, it is likely that some will mistakenly consider AI to be a replacement for human judgment. AI may have—now at least—no way to evaluate the accuracy of its observations or conclusions. Because of this it has been suggested that a product of AI is a *hallucination*.[8] It is critical that users understand the strengths and limitations of these new tools. It is vital that these systems be designed with input from physicians and patients.

It has been proposed that people evaluating the results of AI may be inappropriately trustful. A 2023 report notes that "generative models unilaterally generate confident, fluent responses with no uncertainty representations nor the ability to communicate their absence. This lack of uncertainty signals in generative models could cause greater distortion compared with human inputs."[8] We all have experienced the reality that computers rarely make mistakes. If we ask a computer to do a math problem and get a result which we do not expect, we can assume the question was improperly asked of the computer. We do not ponder the possibility that the computer did it wrong. Because of this lifetime of experience with computer infallibility, we may be improperly trusting of the results of AI.

A pivotal question is how will patients be informed of the results of AI systems? If analysis of an MRI in a forgetful 70-year-old patient suggests that Alzheimer's disease is a likely diagnosis, should this information go directly to the patient? My experience is that radiologists often overinterpret their assessments. It is likely that AI analysis will inherit this tendency. Important information from testing should only be given to the patient by the physician and, hopefully, in person. Input from the physician is necessary to properly understand and place the results in proper context.

AI should help to free up time for doctors to pay attention to patients and should assist with differential diagnosis. It will be desirable if humans can work with computer systems to improve human abilities and not replace them.

References

1. Caplan LR. Paen to physician's patient notes *JAMA Neurol*. 2023;80:7.
2. Astrow AB. On the disenchantment of medicine: Abraham Joshua Heschel's 1964 address to the American Medical Association. *Theor Med Bioeth*. 2018 Dec;39(6):483–97. doi:10.1007/s11017-018-9472-x. PMID: 30411181.
3. Ehrmann DE, Gallant SN, Nagaraj S, Goodfellow SD, Eytan D, Goldenberg A, Mazwi ML. Evaluating and reducing cognitive load should be a priority for machine learning in healthcare. *Nat Med*. 2022 Jul;28(7):1331–3. doi:.1038/s41591-022-01833-z. PMID: 35641825.
4. Bhatt AB, Bae J. Collaborative intelligence to catalyze the digital transformation of healthcare. *NPJ Digit Med*. 2023 Sep 25;6(1):177. doi:10.1038/s41746-023-00920-w. PMID: 37749239; PMCID: PMC10520019.
5. Lee P, Brubeck S, Petro J. Benefits, limits and risks of GPT-4 as an AI chat box for medicine. *N Engl J Med*. 2023;388:12222.
6. Kidd C, Birhane A. How AI can distort human beliefs. *Science*. 2023 Jun 23;380(6651):1222–3. doi:10.1126/science.adi0248. Epub 2023 Jun 22. PMID: 37347992.

7. Bucholc M, James C, Khleifat AA, Badhwar A, Clarke N, Dehsarvi A, Madan CR, Marzi SJ, Shand C, Schilder BM, Tamburin S, Tantiangco HM; Deep Dementia Phenotyping (DEMON) Network; Lourida I, Llewellyn DJ, Ranson JM. Artificial intelligence for dementia research methods optimization. *Alzheimers Dement.* 2023 Aug 28. doi:10.1002/alz.13441. Epub ahead of print. PMID: 37639369.
8. Azamfirei R, Kudchadkar SR, Fackler J. Large language models and the perils of their hallucinations. *Crit Care.* 2023 Mar 21;27(1):120. doi:10.1186/s13054-023-04393-x. PMID: 36945051; PMCID: PMC10032023.

Lesson 36
Do Not Confuse Etiology with Pathophysiology

Pathophysiology describes the processes of disease, and *etiology* presents the cause or causes. Phenylketonuria (PKU) is a relatively common genetic disease which interferes with the metabolism of the amnio acid phenylalanine.[1] The disease is caused by autosomal mutation in the genes for an enzyme which breaks down phenylalanine. The etiology of the disease is genetic. The pathophysiology of the disease describes how excessive phenylalanine causes neuronal death in the brain, causing permanent intellectual disability, seizures, behavioral delay, and psychiatric disorders. Even though the etiology is genetic and repair of defective genes remains difficult, it is possible to treat the disease through a diet low in protein and low in phenylalanine. Early recognition of the gene allows for the diet to be adjusted appropriately to limit the neurological problems. This shows that genetic diseases can have effective environmental treatments.

In 1% of cases of Alzheimer's disease, the disease is caused by an autosomal dominant mutation. In the other 99%, there is no causative gene responsible for the disease. The pathophysiology of the disease involves neuronal proteins amyloid beta and tau and others which are produced in large amounts with abnormal protein structures and poor clearance from the brain. It is commonly assumed that these proteins are the cause of the disease. I believe that it is more appropriate to say that these proteins describe the disease mechanisms (pathophysiology), not the cause (etiology). The etiology of Alzheimer's disease remains unknown in the 99% of cases in which there is not a causative gene.[*]

The most important Alzheimer's disease risk gene is apolipoprotein E.[3] Although it is clear that the Apo E protein is important in the pathophysiology of the disease, it is not the cause. Thus, in persons with two copies of the gene, it is worth asking what important interaction of the gene with some other factor causes the disease. This other factor could be genetic or environmental, of course.[2]

It is important to ask "why" questions (etiology), as well as "how" (pathophysiology) questions. To understand disease, attention to diagnosis, management, and treatment is necessary but not enough. Consideration of the cause is also needed.

---

[*] I have proposed that the disease process in Alzheimer's is initiated by microbial products in the gut.[2]

Do not let etiology decide treatment approaches. It is improper to assume that genetic diseases required genetic treatment. For example, psychotherapy can be valuable in disorders of genetic, environmental, or functional origin. Genetic disease can at times be remedied with nongenetic approaches.

Consider an 81-year-old woman who falls at home and breaks her wrist. In this case, the etiology is clearly traumatic, but the treatment should include consideration of the impact of the fracture on the patient's home life, family dynamics, and medical and mental health. (As well as orthopedic management of the fracture.) That is, there are more things to be considered in this case other than trauma and the broken bone. Did she have osteoporosis? Did she suffer from depression, which increases the risk of falls? Was she malnourished because of loneliness? Clearly there are many factors other than orthopedic repair that are necessary to consider. In this case, the etiology may not be clear (Did she fall because she tripped over a small dog?). The treatment centers around the pathophysiology of the broken bone. But considering etiology and pathophysiology are not enough. The context of the patient's life must also be included in her care.[3]

References

1. Mezzomo TR, Dias MRMG, Santos T, Pereira RM. Dietary intake in individuals with phenylketonuria: An integrative review. *Nutr Hosp.* 2023 Aug 31. doi:10.20960/nh.04579. Epub ahead of print. PMID: 37705455.
2. Friedland RP. Mechanisms of molecular mimicry involving the microbiota in neurodegeneration. *J Alzheimers Dis.* 2015;45(2):349–62. doi:10.3233/JAD-142841. PMID: 25589730.
3. Friedland RP. *Unaging: The Four Factors That Impact How You Age*. Cambridge University Press; 2022.

Lesson 37
Communicate with the Patient

A physician friend of mine visited a cardiologist who convinced him to have a CT scan of coronary calcium deposits to assess his risk of coronary artery disease. The cardiologist called him after the scan, while my friend was with a patient. He told the cardiologist that he was busy and asked if he could speak to him later. The cardiologist then told the friend over the phone that the results of the scan were serious and that he should buy a book about grief so he would be prepared for an early death. This is not how bad news should be communicated.[1] My friend subsequently visited a prominent cardiologist at another hospital and learned that there was no sign whatsoever of abnormal function in his coronary arteries.

It is wrong in almost all cases to give bad news over the telephone. It is important to do it in a private setting in which the patient has enough time to have his questions addressed. Also, the patient should be with family, if feasible. The news should be as truthful as possible but should not be unrealistically pessimistic or alarming. The news must be delivered in an atmosphere of trust, compassion, understanding, and commitment. There must be time for deep listening (Lesson 10) and for the patients' questions to be answered. Nonverbal communication and touching can be helpful. The timing of the interaction should be managed; it is better to develop a relationship with the patient before giving bad news. Patients should also be advised of the possible development of new therapies, and participation in clinical trials may be indicated.[2]

Whenever I inform a patient and family of a diagnosis of Alzheimer's disease I include a discussion of the relative likelihood that the diagnosis is correct. I also make it clear that I am there for them now and throughout the course of their illness. That is, I am not giving them a terminal diagnosis and then informing them to go out and find another doctor. Also, I advise them that the disease is progressive and that truly effective disease-modifying therapies are not currently available. However, there are ways to manage several of the problems that develop with the disease. Also, I tell them that researchers worldwide are intensely investigating the biological mechanisms of the disease and that one day there will be a truly effective therapy available. I advise them that I do not know if that day will be coming in 6 weeks or in 60 years. I try to convey my optimism that the great amount of global work on the disease being done will produce a breakthrough soon.[1]

---

[1] I do not believe that the anti-amyloid beta monoclonal antibodies lecanemab and donanemab are truly disease-modifying.[3]

A new problem has developed regarding communication of bad news. Now many electronic health records have the capacity of sharing laboratory and imaging findings with the patient and family without prior review by the patient's physician. If imaging shows evidence of cancer, the patient should be informed by the physician and not by computer access to the findings. Safeguards must be put in place to protect the communication of findings of major importance via pathways that bypass the physician.

The patient should have the understanding that their questions are welcomed. The ending of a clinic visit should be clear to the patient and family. The physician should not sneak out and wait for the family to ask where he went.

> Time, sympathy and understanding must be lavishly dispensed, but the reward is to be found in that personal bond which forms the greatest satisfaction of the practice of medicine. One of the essential qualities of the clinician is interest in humanity, for the secret of the care of the patient is in caring for the patient.
> —Francis Peabody[4]

Francis Peabody (1881–1927): A Person to Know

Peabody was an American physician and a popular teacher at Harvard Medicine School in Cambridge, Massachusetts. He performed important work on typhoid, poliomyelitis, and pernicious anemia. He was known to be a compassionate physician, dedicating long hours to his patients. His essay on the care of the patient is widely celebrated.[5]

References

1. Harris D, Gilligan T. Delivering bad news. *Med Clin North Am*. 2022 Jul;106(4):641–51. doi:10.1016/j.mcna.2022.02.004. PMID: 35725230.
2. EPEC. *EPEC Education for Physicians Participants Handbook, Module 2, Communicating Bad News*. Robert Wood Johnson Foundation; 2000.
3. Kepp KP, Sensi SL, Johnsen KB, Barrio JR, Høilund-Carlsen PF, Neve RL, Alavi A, Herrup K, Perry G, Robakis NK, Vissel B, Espay AJ. The anti-amyloid monoclonal antibody lecanemab: 16 cautionary notes. *J Alzheimers Dis*. 2023;94(2):497–507. doi:10.3233/JAD-230099. PMID: 37334596.
4. Peabody FW. *The Care of the Patient*. Harvard University Press; 1927.
5. Peabody FW. Landmark article March 19, 1927: The care of the patient. *JAMA* 1984;252:813–8.

Lesson 38
Be Attentive to Medications and Medication Errors

Critical thinking in patient care requires attention to the complexities of drug prescribing and administration. For example, medication errors are common. Errors can include selection of the wrong drug and the wrong dose as well as the wrong patient. Consideration of the ability of the patient to metabolize the drug is necessary. Many patients are taking several medications that interact, with negative effects. *Polypharmacy*, the concurrent use of five or more medications for one or many conditions, is increasingly common. Nearly 50% of older persons are taking one or more drugs that aren't good choices. If a person is taking one drug, there's about a 30% chance they're not taking it properly, and, if they're taking more than five drugs, the risk that they're not taking them properly is very high (poor compliance). You must consider the dynamics of drug binding in the blood. It's important to review all medications and their indications at each visit.[1] If you make changes to medications, it is best to do one at a time, if possible. If you make two changes and the patient does poorly, you may not know which one was responsible.

Remember that patients may not tell you about agents that they take that are available over the counter. It is widely assumed that such substances that can be obtained without prescription are not dangerous. This is incorrect and hazardous. Vitamins A and D are available in pharmacies without prescription but are toxic to the brain at higher doses. An increased risk of bleeding has been observed with several herbs, including chamomile, cranberry, green tea, and others.[2] Furthermore, adverse interactions between herbs and between herbs and drugs can be significant. Herbal products may contain toxic factors including mercury, lead, and arsenic. Furthermore, they may contain none of what is proposed as an active ingredient. In the United States, dietary supplements do not require comprehensive testing or approval from the Food and Drug Administration (FDA). Manufacturers are not required to prove that their products are safe and effective. There are often differences between labeled and actual ingredients or their amounts.

In considering the effects of drugs, remember placebo and nocebo effects (Lessons 29 and 89). Also, most complaints that patients have are capable of resolution by themselves. A person may have a symptom, such as back pain or headache, and find relief with the medication not because of the effect of the agent but because the complaint resolved by itself. A very large proportion of drug effects are due to the fact that most symptoms are temporary. It is important that medications be reviewed regularly and evaluated to determine whether their continuation is necessary.

Consider snake bite. Folk remedies applied in the past for the bite of poisonous snakes included application of gunpowder on the bite and lighting it, use of ammonia, application of a poultice (soft moist mass of bread and clay), whiskey, application of lavender, and many other herbal oils. The reason that there are so many folk treatments for rattlesnake bite is that the bites are rarely fatal. About one-third of bites do not involve delivery of venom, and fewer than 1% of persons bitten by rattlesnakes die from the bite. Similarly, most persons with back pain will get better with rest in a matter of days or weeks. The person who takes an over-the-counter or prescription agent for the pain may falsely attribute their recovery to the therapy.

Many of the most widely used over-the-counter medications for upper respiratory tract infections contain oral phenylephrine. Recently, the FDA has concluded that current scientific data do not support the use of the drug as a nasal decongestant.[3]

One of the first duties of the physician is to educate the masses not to take medicine.

—William Osler

References

1. Friedland RP *Unaging: The Four Factors That Impact How You Age*. University of Cambridge Press; 2022.
2. Tan CSS, Lee SWH. Warfarin and food, herbal or dietary supplement interactions: A systematic review. *Br J Clin Pharmacol*. 2021;87:352–74.
3. FDA. FDA clarifies results of recent advisory committee meeting on oral phenylephrine Sept 14, 2023. https://www.fda.gov/drugs/drug-safety-and-availability/fda-clarifies-results-recent-advisory-committee-meeting-oral-phenylephrine. Accessed Nov 8, 2023.

SECTION IV
CRITICAL THINKING

Lesson 39
Think Deeply (Think Beyond the Obvious)

Our neural networks prepare us for fast decisions. Rapid thinking was essential for survival in the world of our remote ancestors. But rapid thinking is often not enough for important evaluations of what is happening. This lesson presents several examples of how thinking beyond the obvious is critical.

A 72-year-old man falls at home, is taken to the hospital, and is found to have a broken hip. The hip will need to be repaired. What else do we need to know? It is clear that care for the fracture is urgent and cannot be ignored. It is harder to consider the reality behind the situation. Why did he fall? The accident may have been caused by inattention; high or low blood sugar; alcohol; tripping over a small dog, cat, or electrical cord; dizziness; diseases of the ear; medications; cardiac arrhythmia (irregular heartbeat); stroke; depression; drugs; cataracts; or other factors. It's also possible that he was pushed. These considerations are important because the factors responsible for the fall may be a sign of conditions and contextual factors that needs to be recognized. And the events responsible for the fall need to be corrected so he doesn't fall again! And uncovering the cause of the fall may identify an ongoing medical problem that can be remedied.

At the age of 85, an aunt of mine fell down the stairs and had an intracerebral hemorrhage. It was assumed that the hemorrhage was the result of the fall. The incident was witnessed by a neighbor in her building who said that she was standing at the top of the stairs talking to my aunt when my aunt suddenly jumped in the air and fell down the stairs. Clearly, she had had a stroke and the bleed was the cause of the fall, not the other way around.

A distinguished neurologist was receiving an award at an annual meeting of a neurological association. The award came with the opportunity to deliver a plenary lecture to an audience of several thousand neurologists. His talk on stroke followed one on Alzheimer's disease. He started his address by saying that he was glad that he worked on stroke because, unlike Alzheimer's disease, he knows the causes of stroke. He then proceeded to give an excellent speech on the treatment of acute stroke. I did not understand what he meant by saying that he knows the causes of stroke, so I wrote him an email. I congratulated him on his award and asked if he could please explain what the causes of stroke are. He replied saying that strokes are caused by embolism, thrombosis, or hemorrhage. I was shocked to realize that he had not considered what may be the causes of embolism, thrombosis, and hemorrhage. Consider a 68-year-old hypertensive man who has a stroke with thrombosis of the left middle cerebral artery. It is not enough to attribute the stroke to the thrombosis; we need to think more deeply and understand the causes of the thrombosis.*

It is well known that age, smoking, alcoholism, and hypertension are risk factors for stroke. If you have a 78-year-old patient with smoking, alcoholism, and hypertension who has a stroke, can you truthfully say that the reason he had the stroke was because of his age, hypertension, and smoking? What if this patient had an 80-year-old brother who also had hypertension and was smoking but did not have a stroke? Would we be surprised by this? No, we would not be surprised, because **risk factors are not causative**. There must be something else with which the risk factors are interacting to cause disease. These other forces may, of course, be environmental or genetic.

My hope is that questioning will go beyond simple explanations. Consider this question: Why do some people have a stroke involving the left side of the brain and others have the right side affected? Embolic strokes may differ right to left because of the pattern of blood flow in the aortic arch, but I'm not aware of any existing theory as to why hemorrhagic or thrombotic strokes should develop on one side and not the other. Of course, occurrence on the right or left may be random (stochastic). I do not prefer explanations which postulate random factors because often things which are thought to be random appear later to have a nonrandom basis. I propose that left- or right-sided stroke occurs because of the influence of the microbiota (bacteria, fungi, viruses, and other microbes) which reside in the mouth, throat, sinuses, and nose. With my colleagues in Japan we have demonstrated a role of oral bacteria on hemorrhagic stroke in animals and humans.[1] Considerable evidence exists to show the possible pathways by which microbes can influence inflammation in the brain to cause stroke.[2]. Periodontitis, the most common bacterial infection in the mouth, is known to be a risk factor for stroke. Could the laterality of stroke be linked to the laterality of bacterial infections in the mouth?

It is easy to attribute conditions to obvious causes that are often false. For much of the past hundred years following Alois Alzheimer's original report in 1907, it was assumed that severe memory loss in older persons, which was called "senile dementia," "senile psychosis," or "senility," was caused by aging. This error neglected to consider the truth that as many as 40–50% of people at age 100 do not have dementia.

Continuing on the theme of obvious ideas that are false, bed rest was widely advised for patients with coronary heart disease until the past 40 years. It was believed that physical activity would stress the heart, leading to more damage caused by problems with the heart's circulation. It is now known that physical activity is critical for lowering the risk of pulmonary embolism and that clinical status and survival is enhanced by getting patients out of bed as soon as possible. Nobel laureate Dr. Bernard Lown discusses this important development in the management of

---

* A *thrombosis* occurs when the flow of blood in a vessel is blocked because of a clot; an *embolism* occurs when a clot travels from one area to another and blocks the flow of blood; and a *hemorrhage* occurs when a vessel breaks and blood leaves the vessel.

heart disease in his excellent book *The Lost Art of Healing: Practicing Compassion in Medicine*.[3]

There is a story that when new helmets were introduced into the US Army the number of people with facial wounds increased markedly. It was suggested that the helmets were dangerous and should be recalled. However, it was pointed out that the reason that facial wounds were increasing was that people with head injuries were not dying as much as before. Because fewer people died, there were more soldiers who had survived their head wounds.

In the 1960s, the new field of neuroepidemiology uncovered a relationship between the risk of multiple sclerosis (MS) and geographical distance from the Equator. It was found that the disease is more common in northern than southern locations in Europe, North America, and Asia. Also, the disease was found to be particularly uncommon in Africa. Many theories were proposed to explain the geographical effect. One idea suggested that MS was caused by a virus similar to distemper, which is found in dogs, and there are more dogs in the north than in the south. Another theory posited that MS was caused by an immune reaction to wool, as people in the north wear more woolen garments than those in the south. Both theories were investigated and found to be lacking in support.

Can you think of another reason why MS is more common in northern than southern locations?

It was not until 1997 that the idea was presented that the difference was because greater sun exposure in the south causes higher levels of vitamin D in the body. Vitamin D has been known to play an important role in the immune system, and MS is an autoimmune disease.[4] Recently, considerable basic science and clinical studies have shown that vitamin D plays a role in the development of MS. The suggestion that the geographical variation of its incidence was related to sun exposure and vitamin D levels could have been made 30 years earlier if anyone had thought of it. (In 1998, there were two publications on vitamin D and MS; 2010, there were 41.)

I recall being fascinated by the geographical differences in MS occurrence. Most likely I did not think of this relationship myself because I knew so little about vitamins. It was my mistake that, early in my medical education, I focused my efforts narrowly on neurology. (I hope I am alleviating this disability of mine with my current work.)

In Alzheimer's disease, there is reduced metabolism as well as reduced blood flow in the cortex of the brain. It is widely believed that the lowered metabolism and blood flow in the brain is a result of neuronal degeneration. A class of drugs called nootropics has been widely used for the disease. Nootropics are intended to enhance intelligence by increasing the utilization of glucose and oxygen in the brain and increasing blood flow. Evidence that the reduced metabolism and blood flow is causing the disease is lacking. In addition, evidence of therapeutic improvement in dementia with nootropics is absent.[5] Despite this problem with the mechanism of action and the lack of clinical evidence, these drugs have been widely used around the world for decades. The metabolic deficit in Alzheimer is a sign of the neurodegeneration and not a cause.

Thinking deeply requires you to determine what is the fundamental issue in a medical or scientific question. Consider this scenario: a splinter in your foot has caused an infection in the skin with pain, redness, swelling, fever, and increased heart rate. All of these signs of the disease can be helped with an ice pack. However, cooling will not treat the main problem, which is the presence in the body of pathogenic bacteria. The pain, redness, swelling, fever, and increased heart rate caused by an infected splinter are signs of the infection, not the cause. In every clinical and scientific issue, it is worth considering what is fundamental and what is not fundamental.[†] Studies of fundamental matters are more rewarding than are studies of peripheral concerns.

In 1967, the development of microsurgery led to a new procedure to provide additional blood supply to the brain in patients with cerebrovascular disease. It was believed that surgically connecting the external carotid circulation to that of the brain's large vessels, such as the middle cerebral artery, would provide additional blood flow for patients with carotid artery stenosis or occlusion or intracranial vessel narrowing. The procedure was widely performed in thousands of patients worldwide. A large randomized controlled trial, published in 1985, showed that the surgery was not effective in improving patient outcomes.[6] The procedure is not commonly performed today because its efficacy has not been demonstrated. The cerebral circulation is not like the pipes in a building. More blood flow may not help if the increased flow is not available to the neurons on the capillary level.

The history of medicine is made up extensively of stories like these. It is necessary to go beyond apparently obvious causes to think more deeply and not be biased by preconceived ideas.

The foolish look at events, the wise look at causes.
—Attributed to Gautama Buddha[7]

References

1. Ikeda S, Saito S, Hosoki S, Tonomura S, Yamamoto Y, Ikenouchi H, Ishiyama H, Tanaka T, Hattori Y, Friedland RP, Carare RO, Kuriyama N, Yakushiji Y, Hara H, Koga M, Toyoda K, Nomura R, Takegami M, Nakano K, Ihara M. Harboring Cnm-expressing Streptococcus mutans in the oral cavity relates to both deep and lobar cerebral microbleeds. *Eur J Neurol*. 2023 Nov;30(11):3487–96. doi:10.1111/ene.15720. Epub 2023 Feb 16. PMID: 36708081.
2. Tonomura S, Ihara M, Friedland RP. Microbiota in cerebrovascular disease: A key player and future therapeutic target. *J Cereb Blood Flow Metab*. 2020 Jul;40(7):1368–80. doi:10.1177/0271678X20918031. Epub 2020 Apr 20. PMID: 32312168; PMCID: PMC7308516.
3. Lown B. *The Lost Art of Healing: Practicing Compassion in Medicine*. Ballantine Books; 1999.
4. Gandhi F, Jhaveri S, Avanthika C, Singh A, Jain N, Gulraiz A, Shah P, Nasir F. Impact of vitamin D supplementation on multiple sclerosis. *Cureus*. 2021 Oct 5;13(10):e18487. doi:10.7759/cureus.18487. PMID: 34754649; PMCID: PMC8567111.

[†] "Fundamental" is defined as "Serving as a basis or foundation; ... forming an essential or indispensable part of a system" (Oxford English Dictionary).

5. Olin J, Schneider L, Novit A, Luczak S. Hydergine for dementia. *Cochrane Database Syst Rev.* 2001;2:CD000359. doi:10.1002/14651858.CD000359. PMID: 11405961.
6. Holohan TV. Extracranial-intracranial bypass to reduce the risk of ischemic stroke. *CMAJ.* 1991 Jun 1;144(11):1457–65. PMID: 2032198; PMCID: PMC1335677.
7. Kornfield J. *A Path with Heart: A Guide Through the Perils and Promises of a Spiritual Life.* Bantam; 1993.

Lesson 40
How Often Do Rare Events Occur?

It is tempting to say that, by definition, rare events occur rarely. We can imagine certain rare events and recall that they do not happen frequently. For example, hail the size of 1 centimeter is rarely observed (I have never seen it myself). **The reality is that it is only individual rare events that occur rarely. The more significant fact is that everything that happens is a rare event, and rare events happen commonly (all the time!).** Imagine a patient with migraine who comes to clinic (migraine is a common cause of headache). If we consider the patient's background in depth, considering her age, education, medical history, occupation, medications, and genetics, we can be sure that such a medical visit has never occurred before. There are, of course, similarities from one person to another, but if the situation is investigated with sufficient complexity, it is apparent that each patient visit is a rare event.

Another way to consider this is to realize that each grain of rice is unique, and there are no grains of rice anywhere on earth that are identical to other grains. Of course, they all have many similarities, but if we consider their microscopic three-dimensional structure, we can appreciate that there cannot be two grains of rice that are identical on an ultrastructural level.

I recall being astounded as a child by the phenomenon that all snowflakes have a different configuration. (It is impossible for two snowflakes to form complicated patterns in the same way. Scientists estimate that there are up to 10^{158} snowflake possibilities. That's 10^{70} times more configurations than there are atoms in the universe.[1]) What I did not realize was that this situation of uniqueness was universal. Charles Darwin also observed that no two barnacles of the same species are identical.[2]

This point of view is important for understanding the distinctiveness of each patient. A pediatrician may see tens of patients a day, all having a runny nose, low-grade fever, and earache. Most, or possibly all, may have ear infections, perhaps requiring pain medications, decongestants, and antibiotics. Critically, the doctor must be aware that patients with a runny nose, low-grade fever, and earache may also have meningitis, requiring urgent evaluation and management. The pediatrician cannot be deluded into believing that her patients are all the same.

Another aspect of the fact that rare events happen frequently is the realization that although individual rare diseases are not common, they do occur. I have found that many physicians have a bias against considering rare diseases because of the erroneous belief that they don't occur. This is a result, of course, of a bias of clinical experience. If a doctor has been practicing for 40 years and has never seen a certain condition, he may mistakenly assume that it doesn't happen. Similarly, many radiological and surgical procedures have low rates of complications. Although these complications do not occur frequently, it is a mistake to think that they don't happen.

I am aware of a case in which a healthy 56-year-old woman underwent back surgery for intervertebral disc disease. Tragically, the neurosurgeon's hand slipped in putting a screw in the spine and the aorta was ruptured, leading to her death. A 20-year-old college baseball pitcher died in 2021 during elbow surgery because of improper placement of the endotracheal tube (a tube placed between the vocal cords through the trachea allowing for ventilation of the lungs). These two tragedies are very infrequent complications of surgery, but the risk of their occurrence is greater than zero.

It is also necessary to be aware that some things are so rare that they have not yet occurred. The HIV/AIDS pandemic began in the 1980s as a largely unprecedented event. Another extraordinary event was noted in 1976, when a 23-year-old graduate student in chemistry had the sudden onset of what appeared to be Parkinson's disease. Rapid onset of the disease in a young person had never been noted previously.[3] (The neurotoxic nature of his illness is discussed in Lesson 93.) It is the responsibility of clinicians and scientists to be aware that some events may have never happened before.[4] It is necessary to recognize truly novel situations when they develop. The "black swan" event is something which is unpredictable and so rare that it has never happened (Lesson 46).

Consider a rare condition, Creutzfeldt-Jakob disease. The incidence and prevalence of the disease is about 1 per million worldwide (the incidence and prevalence are the same because the average survival is about 1 year.) If you live in an area with a population of 10 million, you can expect 10 people to have the disease at any one time in the area. It is certainly an error to think you will not be seeing one of these patients yourself.

It is often said in medicine that "when you hear hoofbeats you should think of horses not zebras." This is often wise advice. However, your choices should depend on the situation. If you are in the savanna in Kenya and hear hoofbeats, it may very well be zebras (or possibly wildebeest, antelope, or other hoofed savannah dwellers).*

It is widely recommended to follow the advice of *Occam's razor*. That is, the simplest explanation for phenomena is usually best. If a patient has abnormal physical signs which can be explained by a single disease, it may be best to favor that choice as the cause rather than postulating that the patient has two, three, or more different diseases. The term "razor" is applied to indicate the shaving away of unnecessary assumptions. The principle has been credited to William of Ockham (1285–1348) who said, "plurality must never be posited without necessity." A similar sentiment was stated by Isaac Newton: "We are to admit to no more causes of natural things than such as are both true and sufficient to explain their appearances." However, it is not uncommon that applying Occam's razor and Newton's logic leads to erroneous conclusions. Unfortunately, having one disease is usually not protective against

---

* Consider the question, how many zebras are there in Canada? The answer is not zero because zebras can be found in zoos and parks.

having any other one. It is important to have an open mind and be aware of the risks of accepting the simplest explanation. Occam's razor may be fine for barbers—but it may lead diagnosticians astray.

> The disease is common; the patient is unique.
> —Abraham Joshua Heschel[5]

References

1. Stempien A. Are all snowflakes really different? The science of winter. Smithsonian Science Education Center. https://ssec.si.edu/stemvisions-blog/are-all-snowflakes-really-different-science-winter
2. Sacks O. *On the Move: A Life*. Knopf; 2015.
3. Langston JW. The MPTP story. *J Parkinsons Dis*. 2017;7(s1):S11–S19. doi:10.3233/JPD-179006.
4. Taleb N. *The Black Swan, Second Edition: The Impact of the Highly Improbable*. Random House; 2019.
5. Heschel AJ. *The Insecurity of Freedom*. Henry Regnery Company; 1963.

Lesson 41
Do Not Depend on Logic Alone

Logic is defined as "reasoning conducted or assessed according to strict principles of validity" (Oxford Languages online). We are taught throughout our years of education to think logically. This long experience of the importance of logic obscures the great depth of our imagination. The Bengali poet Rabindranath Tagore felt that logic alone was not enough. He said, "A mind all logic is like a knife all blade. It makes the hand bleed that uses it."[1]

The idea that nonrational factors can contribute to creativity was proposed by the fourth-century BC Greek philosopher Plato, who was a student of Socrates. The German philosopher Friedrich Nietzsche thought that dreams were the source of his creative principle. The British poet Coleridge reported that an opium dream led to the creation of his poem *Kubla Khan*. Robert Louis Stevenson noted that several of his novels had plots originating in dreams.

There are numerous stories in the history of science of discoveries resulting from nonlogical mental processes. The neurophysiologist Otto Loewi (1873–1961), who discovered the first neurotransmitter, acetylcholine, devised an experiment on the electrical conduction of nervous impulses while dreaming. According to Loewi, "The night before Easter Sunday (1920) I awoke, turned on the light and jotted down a few notes on a tiny slip of thin paper. Then I fell asleep again. It occurred to me at 6.00 o'clock in the morning that during the night I had written down something important, but I was unable to decipher the scrawl. The next night, at 3.00 o'clock, the idea returned. It was the design of an experiment to determine whether or not the hypothesis of chemical transmission that I had uttered 17 years ago was correct. I got up immediately, went to the laboratory, and performed a simple experiment on a frog heart according to the nocturnal design."[1]

The French mathematician Henri Poincare experienced sudden insights at times of relaxation which led him to important advances in his work.[2] He said "Often when one works at a hard question, nothing good is accomplished at the first attack. Then one takes a rest, longer or shorter, and sits down anew to the work ... when all of a sudden the decisive idea presents itself to the mind. It might be said that the conscious work has been more fruitful because it has been interrupted and the rest has given back to the mind its force and freshness."

---

[1] Tagore won the Nobel Prize in Literature in 1913.

August Kekulé (1829–1896) was a Belgian organic chemist trying to understand the structure of benzene. While daydreaming he had an image of a snake biting its own tail, which led him to come up with the correct structure of a hexagon for benzene, having six carbons in a circle (a benzene ring).[3]

The mind is a powerful tool. You may solve an important problem by concentrating your attention. You may also find that the problem is resolved spontaneously without your attention. New approaches to the problem may be found through relaxation without concentrated attention. Important insight may spontaneously alight upon the branches of your imagination. It is important to be open to the potential for such a development. It is wise, as recommended by Sir William Osler, to have with you at all times a little notebook which you can use to jot down such apparently random thoughts that may be of interest. The history of science is filled with stories of great insights that were the product of relaxation and not concentration. Mediation is a valuable method of allowing the mind to clear so new ideas can develop.

Clearly relaxation-induced insights are not enough. Real work is also required.

If you go on hammering away at a problem, it seems to get tired, lies down and lets you catch it.
—W. L. Bragg, Australian Nobel laureate in physics (the youngest ever, having received the award at age 25)[4]

No-one ever said that science is logical. Oh, everyone says that science is logical, but it's not true. After all, it is done by people and people are notoriously illogical.
—James Peebles, Physics Nobel laureate, 2019[5]

Otto Loewi (1873–1961): A Person to Know

Loewi was a German pharmacologist who discovered that nerve impulses can be transmitted through molecules. He identified acetylcholine as an endogenous (internal) neurotransmitter and received the 1936 Nobel Prize in Physiology or Medicine with his friend Sir Henry Dale.[1] His work was important in understanding the physiology of the sympathetic nervous system.

References

1. McCoy AN, Tan SY. Otto Loewi (1873–1961): Dreamer and Nobel laureate. *Singapore Med J.* 2014 Jan;55(1):3–4. doi:10.11622/smedj.2014002. PMID: 24452970; PMCID: PMC4291908.
2. Poincare H. Mathematical creation. 1904. The Foundations of Science: Science and Hypothesis, the Value of Science. Science and Method. https://www.gutenberg.org/files/39713/39713-h/39713-h.htm.

3. Rothenberg A. Creative cognitive processes in Kekulé's discovery of the structure of the benzene molecule. *Am J Psychol.* Autumn 1995;108(3):419–38.
4. Perutz M. *Science Is Not a Quiet Life: Unraveling the Atomic Mechanism of Haemoglobin.* Imperial College Press; 1997: 65.
5. Physics World. James Peebles: A life in cosmology. *Physics World.* Jun 2, 2023. https://physicsworld.com/a/james-peebles-a-life-in-cosmology/.

Lesson 42
Although Intuition Cannot Replace Evidence, It Can Be Valuable

Intuition: An ability to understand or know something immediately based on your feelings rather than facts.
—Cambridge Dictionary

Empirical: Based on what is experienced or seen rather than on theory.
—Cambridge Dictionary

It is important to consider the insights that may come to you when you are asleep, daydreaming, or otherwise not devoted actively to thought (Lesson 41). At the same time the insights received need to be evaluated with evidence. Intuition is not enough.

Aristotle (384–322 BC), the influential Greek philosopher and teacher of Alexander the Great, had a profound influence on Western thought. He preferred to rely upon intuition rather than evidence to answer questions about the world. Most famously he believed that women had fewer teeth than men. He did not trouble himself to look for himself to see if he was correct. He thought that his analysis of the matter did not need verification with evidence. We all would hope that such a mistaken strategy would have been extinguished by the growth of science in the past several hundred years. Unfortunately, this is not the case.

I had a neurologist colleague who preferred using two drugs for new-onset epilepsy in adults. I asked him why he didn't use the preferred method, which at the time had shown that a single new drug was more effective than the two he was using. He said he preferred his two drugs because one inhibited the electrical activity from beginning and the other inhibited its spread in the brain. It was clear that he preferred his idea over evidence, to the detriment of his patients.

A modern story about the danger of reliance upon intuition and not data concerns a new drug for Alzheimer's disease (Lesson 45).

While I propose that intuition cannot replace evidence, it is critical to realize that intuition can provide valuable insights. The cerebral cortex of man contains more than 100 billion neurons in each hemisphere, and each one may be connected to 10,000 others. A recent contribution called "the largest map of the human brain ever made" showed that the brain has more than 3,000 different types of cells.[1] Lots of things can go on in this magnificent assembly that do not reach consciousness!

Intuition cannot be relied upon alone, especially if conclusions are not supported by evidence. At the same time, we need to be open to the possibility that intuition may aid understanding in profound ways.

> The best logic for a particular science abandons the rules of logic when it begins serious discourse.... Wanting to make practical use of logic is like consulting the field of mechanics before learning to walk.
> —Arthur Schopenhauer, German philosopher (1788–1860)

> [R]ules and forms of logic are not enough to produce an ingenious thought.
> —Rudolf Eucken, German philosopher (1846–1926)

> Slowly we crept upstream ... laboriously feeling—it was the dry season—for the channels between the sandbanks. Lost in thought I sat on the deck of the barge, struggling to find the elementary and universal conception of the ethical which I had not discovered in any philosophy. Sheet after sheet I covered with disconnected sentences, merely to keep myself concentrated on the problem. Late on the third day, at the very moment when, at sunset, we were making our way through a herd of hippopotamuses, there flashed upon my mind, unforeseen and unsought, t—he phrase, "Reverence for Life." The iron door had yielded: the path in the thicket had become visible. Now I had found my way to the idea in which world- and life-affirmation and ethics are contained side-by-side! Now I knew that the world-view of ethical world- and life-affirmation, together with its ideals of civilization, is founded in thought.
> —Albert Schweitzer (1875–1965)[2]

Albert Schweitzer (1875–1965): A Person to Know

Schweitzer was an Alsatian physician, a theologian, a musicologist, and a humanitarian. Winner of the 1952 Nobel Peace Prize for his philosophy of "reverence for life," he founded a hospital in French Equatorial Africa, now Gabon. His wife served as his nurse and anesthetist, and together they organized the building of the hospital, where he died. Although he was an opponent of colonialism, he was accused of paternalism in his attitude toward Africans.[3]

References

1. Conroy G. This is the largest map of the human brain ever made. *Nature*. 2023 Oct 12. doi:10.1038/d41586-023-03192-2. Epub ahead of print. PMID: 37828214.
2. Schweitzer A. *Out of My Life and Thought*, trans. C. T. Campion. Beacon Press; 1948: 184–6.
3. Schweitzer A. *The Philosophy of Civilization*. Prometheus Books; 1987.

Lesson 43
Should You Think Out of the Box?

Thinking "out of the box" is a metaphor for thinking in an unconventional manner, with creativity. The idea may have originated in the nine-dot puzzle, which can only be solved by linking the nine dots using four straight lines so they connect outside of the "box."[1]

Many persons first attempting the puzzle assume, incorrectly, that the lines must be completely inside the dimensions of the nine dots. Actually, there is no such limit and the puzzle cannot be solved without going outside of the imaginary box. The main point is that we often limit our imagination by assuming there are more rules than are actually present.

Thinking outside the box involves two concepts: (1) there is a box that can restrict our thinking, and (2) we can do our thinking outside the limits of the box. **I prefer a single concept: that there is no box.** Human creativity should not be limited by any geometrical formation or other restrictions which impair creativity and imagination.

There are countless examples of scientific advances that have come about because of respect for the importance of the freedom of thought. Consider the development of the radioimmunoassay by Roslyn Yalow and Solomon Berson (1918–1972). The method uses antibodies to measure the amount of an antigen in a biological sample. The use of antibodies in a biological assay was an innovative and pioneering approach. The method is extraordinarily sensitive and helpful in a wide range of clinical questions. Yalow won the 1977 Nobel Prize in Physiology or Medicine for the development of the technique. (Yalow was the second woman to win the prize. Dr. Berson died before the prize was awarded.)

In a paper recording her Nobel address, published in *Science* in 1978, Dr. Yalow included a copy of a letter of rejection from the *Journal of Clinical Investigation* (1955).[2] In the letter, the journal's editor states that the reviewers could not allow publication because they did not believe that the binding protein was an antibody.

Rosalyn Yalow (1921–2011): A Person to Know

Dr. Yalow went to Hunter College in New York City, taking advantage of free tuition. In her Nobel biography, she thanks her high school chemistry teacher. She originally went to business school to learn stenography but obtained a physics position at the University of Illinois.* At the Bronx Veterans Administration Medical Center her laboratory was initially in the janitor's closet. As she studied the antibody binding of insulin she and Berson realized that it could be a tool for measuring circulating small peptides.[3] The US National Library of Medicine has nearly 100,000 papers concerning radioimmunoassay.

> The world cannot afford the loss of the talents of half its people if we are to solve the many problems which beset us.
> —Roslyn Yalow, Nobel Prize acceptance speech

> Imagination is more important than knowledge.
> —Albert Einstein

References

1. Kitch B. How to encourage thinking outside the box Jan 20, 2023. Mural. https://www.mural.co/blog/think-outside-the-box.
2. Yalow RS. Radioimmunoassay: A probe for the fine structure of biologic systems. *Science*. 1978 Jun 16;200(4347):1236–45. doi: 0.1126/science.208142. PMID: 208142.
3. Yalow R. Biographical essay, Nobel Prize in Physiology or Medicine. https://www.nobelprize.org/prizes/medicine/1977/yalow/biographical/

---

* She was the only woman among 400 members of the College of Engineering. She got a A-minus grade in a physics class and her professor said that this showed that women cannot do physics.

Lesson 44
All Models Are Wrong

> All models are wrong; the practical question is how wrong do they have to be to not be useful.
> —George E. P. Box (1919–2013), British statistician

Animal models can provide critical insights into human disease. The details of experimentation involving animal models must be carefully considered to be as close as possible to the human condition. Let's consider how mice are used for studies of spinal cord injury.

The animals are anesthetized and a laminectomy performed so that the spinal cord is exposed (the back portion of the vertebrae are removed).[1] A quantified physical trauma is then delivered directly to the cord. Researchers tell me that the model using the surgically exposed cord is best because it is "cleanest" and most reproducible. However, this model is creating an injury that will never ever occur in people. The model could more precisely mimic the human condition by having the weight dropped on the intact vertebral column with intact skin in an anaesthetized mouse.

In human spinal cord injury, the traumatized cord is exposed to the broken bones of the vertebrae and dirt, clothing, and other irritants. The broken bones also contain bone marrow, which will influence immune reactions to the injury. An important component of spinal cord injury are the secondary factors that extend the primary injury and worsen the deficit. Corticosteroids were studied for acute spinal cord injury in the 1960s, with the thought that their reduction of edema will be helpful.* Animal studies in mice and dogs demonstrated the beneficial effect of steroids on spinal cord injury. However, large studies of the effect of corticosteroids on acute spinal cord injury in humans showed no difference in neurological improvement, and steroid treatment had several serious side effects. I propose that the different mechanisms of injury in mice and humans may be responsible for varying experimental results in treatment trials. I suggest that it is more important for the animal model to closely mimic the human condition and less important for it to be reproducible.

Mouse models of human genetic conditions have been widely utilized to study molecular mechanisms of disease. The unique characteristics of mouse models has not always been considered. Compared to humans, mice have a faster metabolic rate and different dietary requirements, lipid metabolism, and glucose transport, And, of

---

* Steroids have neuroprotective effects with improved blood flow, prevention of calcium accumulation, and inhibition of inflammation.

course, mice are nocturnal and capable of hibernation. Also, the lifetime of a mouse is much shorter than that of a person. Thus, it would not be surprising if the phenotypical effects of the mutation are different in mice and humans. (A *phenotype* refers to an observable trait; *genotype* is the genetic makeup of an organism.) All of the differences between the rodent model and the human condition need to be considered.

After the discovery of the autosomal dominant mutations responsible for early-onset Alzheimer's disease in the late 1980s, researchers around the world began developing transgenic mice that harbor one or more copies of the mutations. The fact that only 1% of Alzheimer's disease cases is caused by a mutation has not slowed down the extensive dedication to mouse models of the disease. According to the US National Library of Medicine there are 16,127 papers on transgenic mice and Alzheimer's disease (July, 2024). Despite all this work we still do not have a truly effective disease-modifying therapy for the disease.[2]

Nobel laureate Albert Szent-Györgyi had a lot to say about the choice of model systems (Lesson 68).

It is important for disease models to replicate the human condition as much as possible. Work with animal models must carefully consider the unique features of each model.

References

1. Saraswat Ohri S, Andres KR, Howard RM, Brown BL, Forston MD, Hetman M, Whittemore SR. Acute pharmacological inhibition of protein kinase R-like endoplasmic reticulum kinase signaling after spinal cord injury spares oligodendrocytes and improves locomotor recovery. *J Neurotrauma*. 2023 May;40(9–10):1007–19. doi:10.1089/neu.2022.0177. Epub 2023 Jan 25. PMID: 36503284; PMCID: PMC10162120.
2. Kepp KP, Sensi SL, Johnsen KB, Barrio JR, Høilund-Carlsen PF, Neve RL, Alavi A, Herrup K, Perry G, Robakis NK, Vissel B, Espay AJ. The anti-amyloid monoclonal antibody lecanemab: 16 cautionary notes. *J Alzheimers Dis*. 2023;94(2):497–507. doi: 10.3233/JAD-230099. PMID: 37334596.

Lesson 45
Biomarkers Are Not the Disease Itself

In June 2021, the US Food and Drug Administration (FDA) granted accelerated approval to aducanumab, a monoclonal antibody designed for the treatment of Alzheimer's disease. Randomized placebo-controlled studies demonstrated that the antibody helped remove amyloid deposits in the brain. These amyloid plaques have been an important finding in the disease for more than 120 years. However, the drug did not improve the rate of cognitive decline, and more than 40% of research participants experienced potentially hazardous side effects involving bleeding or swelling in the brain. An FDA advisory panel voted 10 to 0 that the antibodies should not be approved. The failure of aducanumab to help the patient followed similar results from crenazemab, another monoclonal antibody.

Janet Woodcock, the FDA commissioner who approved aducanumab despite the objection of the advisory panel defended her decision, saying, "Fundamentally, at some point, the 50-year investment in basic science has to merge with clinical methodology and we have to just stop thinking empirical evaluation is the only way of evaluating truth."[1] *Empirical evaluation* is making judgments based on observation and experience rather than on theory or logic. I was astounded to see an FDA Commisioner admit her distrust of evidence.

The FDA's decision was supported by several leading investigators in the Alzheimer field as well as by the US Alzheimer's Association. They were recommending the approval of the drug despite the fact that it did not help the patient.[2] It is remarkable how they were misguided by the focus on biomarker effects. The reduction of amyloid plaque in the brain is a biomarker. But it is a mistake to use a drug that affects only biomarkers and not the welfare of the patient.

An example of the nature of biomarkers may be the use of aspirin for a sore throat caused by a *Streptococcus* infection. Aspirin will relieve the pain and redness and reduce the fever, but it will not help to destroy the bacteria causing the pharyngitis. The amyloid plaques removed by the monoclonal antibody are a marker of the disease, not the disease itself. The approval of aducanumab despite its lack of efficacy led to one of the least successful drug launches in the history of the US pharmaceutical industry.

In July 2023, a diagnostic service announced a plasma amyloid beta protein test for Alzheimer's disease that will be available for anyone over 18 years of age.[3] The test, which will cost $399, will be sold as a direct-to-consumer Alzheimer's disease blood test. Particularly concerning is the fact that the specificity of the test is relatively low. (*Specificity* is the degree to which a diagnostic test is specific for a particular disease or trait.) As it is available directly to consumers, it is likely to be frequently misunderstood. For example, an 80-year-old person who has the test may have an indication of an Alzheimer process going on, but it might be a process which will not affect her in her lifetime. Furthermore, many people will have the test without having a comprehensive evaluation. Laboratory tests should not be allowed to replace the guidance of a physician.

References

1. Brennan Z. Woodcock defends Biogen's new Alzheimer's drug, says it has more supportive data than many past accelerated approvals. Endpoint news. Jun 22, 2021. https://endpts.com/woodcock-defends-biogens-new-alzheimers-drug-says-it-has-more-supportive-data-than-many-past-accelerated-approvals/.
2. Rizk JG, Lewin JC. FDA's dilemma with the aducanumab approval: Public pressure and hope, surrogate markers and efficacy, and possible next steps. *BMJ Evid Based Med.* 2023 Apr;28(2):78–82. doi:10.1136/bmjebm-2022-111914. Epub 2022 Apr 21. PMID: 35450946.
3. ALZ Forum. Direct-to-consumer Alzheimer's blood test opens Pandora's box. Aug 31, 2023. https://www.alzforum.org/news/community-news/direct-consumer-alzheimers-blood-test-opens-pandoras-box.

Lesson 46
Absence of Evidence Is Not Evidence of Absence

In the 1990s, my colleagues and I published a series of papers showing the role of lifestyle factors, including diet and cognitive activity at home and at work, on the risk of Alzheimer's disease.[1] Others had shown the influence of hypertension, diabetes, hyperlipidemia, and tobacco use with increased Alzheimer's disease risk. A 2010 "State of the Science Conference" statement on preventing Alzheimer's disease and cognitive decline said that because the "quality of evidence was low for all of these associations" they were unable to draw firm conclusions on the association of any modifiable factor with the risk of the disease.[2] A similar conclusion was reached by the US National Academies of Science, Engineering and Medicine in 2017.[3] I felt that these decisions were erroneous because "absence of evidence is not evidence of absence."* Obtaining convincing evidence concerning the influence of lifestyle factors on human disease is difficult. It should not be assumed that the interaction does not exist if evidence for it is not satisfying all of the demands for scholarly publication.

Many items sold over the counter are assumed to be safe for human consumption even though they have not been comprehensively tested. This is also true for artificial colors, artificial flavors, and preservatives. Some food-based preservatives are known to be carcinogenic. It is a mistake to assume that these products are safe because we don't have evidence that they are not safe.

There is considerable evidence that alcohol intake by a childbearing mother can have negative effects on the baby. The US Centers for Disease Control recommended a limit of two drinks per day for pregnant women in 1977. It is clearly difficult to document a negative effect of low doses of alcohol on the baby. Even if an effect of low doses cannot be documented, it is reasonable to suggest that alcohol use during pregnancy should be avoided. It is known that the brain of the fetus can be damaged by alcohol. A comprehensive study of dose response relationships of alcohol exposure during pregnancy would need to follow babies for 30 years to examine cognitive capacities and other neurocognitive outcomes. The fact that these studies have not yet been done and will never be done should not imply that alcohol use during pregnancy is safe. In 2018, the recommendations were changed, and it was recommended that there is no known safe amount of alcohol use during pregnancy.[4]

---

* This phrase is often attributed to the astronomer Carl Sagan.

What about caffeine exposure in pregnancy? An epidemiological study in 1983 showed that caffeine consumption during pregnancy is not associated with reduced child growth. This was interpreted by the news media to imply that drinking caffeine during pregnancy was safe for the baby. Why would anyone think that the observation that reduced fetal growth is not linked to caffeine exposure in pregnancy means that caffeine consumption was safe? Caffeine is a potent drug with powerful effects on the central nervous system. It is the most widely used addictive substance in the world. Chronic intrauterine exposure to caffeine may have long-lasting effects on the development of neural systems. The demonstration of no caffeine intake effects on the baby's growth tells us nothing about the possible effects of prenatal caffeine exposure on important structural and functional aspects of brain development.[†]

In legal settings, a defendant will be found not guilty if there is an absence of evidence of guilt. This is because of the presumption of innocence (a defendant in a criminal trial is assumed to be innocent until they have been proved guilty; guilt must be proved beyond a reasonable doubt). It is important to keep in mind that drugs, supplements, vitamins, and natural products are not people, and they are not entitled to presumption of innocence until being proved guilty.

A concept related to "the absence of evidence is not the evidence of absence" is the idea of the *black swan*, as proposed by statistician Nassim Taleb in his book *The Black Swan: The Impact of the Highly Improbable*.[6] A "black swan" is a highly improbable event which is unpredictable and powerful. It is human nature to focus on things we know already and to not consider what we don't know. Furthermore, we often don't consider what we might think of as impossible. People in Europe before the discovery of Australia believed that all swans were white. They believed that black swans did not exist because they had never been seen. However, all that is needed is one single observation of a black swan to invalidate the statement that there are no black swans. Thus, the fact that we have no evidence that black swans do not exist does not mean that they are truly not present. The scenario has been applied to financial crises that were apparently completely unique, such as that of 2008.

The chief message from the black swan concept is the importance of being aware of what you don't know. Don't assume that because something hasn't happened and it's not expected to occur that it won't happen. Also, just because something could be very horrible if it did happen doesn't mean that it won't happen.

Consider neurologist William Langston, who noted several cases of acute onset of Parkinson's disease in 1982[7] (Lesson 46). His study of these cases showed that the persons affected had been poisoned by a novel agent that caused the specific damage to the brainstem nuclei involved in the disease. The presentation of these cases was completely unprecedented, and his investigation was one of the most important scientific advances in twentieth-century neuroscience. We are fortunate that Langston had the courage and tenacity to comprehensively pursue this unprecedented situation.

[†] A more comprehensive recent study has shown that caffeine consumption during pregnancy, even at low levels, is associated with growth retardation.[5]

When we see a patient with a novel presentation we look to our past experience for examples. It is also necessary to be open to the possibility that what you are seeing is something completely novel.

The author of *Black Swan*, Nassim Talleb asks an important question.

What are our minds made for? It looks as if we have the wrong user's manual. Our minds do not seem made to think and introspect; if they were, things would be easier for us today, but then we would not be here today and I would not have been here to talk about it—my counterfactual, introspective, and hard-thinking ancestor would have been eaten by a tiger while his nonthinking, but faster-reacting cousin would have run for cover. Consider that thinking is time-consuming and generally a great waste of energy, that our predecessors spent more than a hundred million years as nonthinking mammals and that in the blip in our history during which we have used our brain we have used it on subjects too peripheral to matter. Evidence shows that we do much less thinking than we believe we do—except, of course, when we think about it.[6]

Consider also the possibility of a white swan event. This is the occurrence of an event that is very likely or certain to occur, which is easy to predict. It is easy to measure what the impact of the white swan event will be. Consider this white swan scenario: a frail older woman has poor blood pressure control, poor blood sugar management, lives alone, and has poor medication compliance (not taking medication in the right dose at the right time). It is highly likely that this woman will fall and that the fall will lead to pneumonia with a significant risk of dying. White swan events are often not recognized by patients, caregivers, family members, and physicians. Denial of white swan events can be deadly (Lesson 33).

> Science is a topography of ignorance.
> —Oliver Wendell Holmes Sr.

Oliver Wendell Holmes Sr. (1809–1894): A Person to Know

Holmes was an American physician, a literary figure, an attorney, and a lecturer. He was the father of Oliver Wendell Holmes Jr., who was a Justice on the US Supreme Court. He advanced the use of the stethoscope and denounced homeopathy. He is noted to have observed that if all medicines were tossed into the sea "it would be better for mankind—and all the worse for the fishes." He supported the role of infectious agents in childbed fever and promoted antisepsis, as later advised by Ignaz Semmelweis (Lesson 34).

References

1. Friedland RP. *Unaging: The Four Factors That Impact How You Age*. University of Cambridge Press; 2022.
2. Daviglus ML, Bell CC, Berrettini W, Bowen PE, Connolly ES Jr, Cox NJ, Dunbar-Jacob JM, Granieri EC, Hunt G, McGarry K, Patel D, Potosky AL, Sanders-Bush E, Silberberg D, Trevisan M. NIH state-of-the-science conference statement: Preventing Alzheimer's disease and cognitive decline. *NIH Consens State Sci Statements*. 2010 Apr 28;27(4):1–30. PMID: 20445638.
3. National Academies of Sciences, Engineering, and Medicine; Division of Behavioral and Social Sciences and Education; Board on Behavioral, Cognitive, and Sensory Sciences. *Understanding Pathways to Successful Aging: Behavioral and Social Factors Related to Alzheimer's Disease: Proceedings of a Workshop–in Brief*. National Academies Press (US); 2017 Sep 28. PMID: 28976725.
4. Centers for Disease Control and Prevention. Fetal alcohol spectrum disorders (FASDs). Mar 25, 2018. https://www.cdc.gov/ncbddd/fasd/alcohol-use.html.
5. Mills JL, Holmes LB, Aarons JH, Simpson JL, Brown ZA, Jovanovic-Peterson LG, Conley MR, Graubard BI, Knopp RH, Metzger BE. Moderate caffeine use and the risk of spontaneous abortion and intrauterine growth retardation. *JAMA*. 1993 Feb 3;269(5):593–7. PMID: 8421363.
6. Taleb N. *The Black Swan: The Impact of the Highly Improbable* (2nd ed.). Random House; 2019.
7. Langston JW, Palfreman J. *The Case of the Frozen Addicts* (2nd ed.). Pantheon Books; 2014. ISBN 978-1-61499-331-5.

Lesson 47
Being Wrong (at Times) Is OK

Although science has made great advances in the past 50 years or so, it is clearer than ever that there is so much that we don't know. Every scientific advance comes along with a plethora of questions. The first step in understanding a scientific problem is appreciating what you don't know and designing questions to address your ignorance. The same progress applies to the evaluation of your patients—you must be aware of what you don't know to decide how to proceed.

As you analyze scientific and patient-centered questions it is inevitable that there will be times when you are wrong. This is not necessarily a bad thing. Errors can often lead to progress. This principle is best expressed by Claude Bernard, who said "**Theories are not true or false, they are fertile or sterile.**" Bernard was a great physiologist who elucidated the process of glucose metabolism in the liver. In his book, *An Introduction to the Study of Experimental Medicine* (1865), he remarked how happy he was to have his ideas proved to be incorrect because that meant that he had learned something.[1,*]

It is reported that when Albert Einstein was found to be wrong, he was delighted because he felt that he had learned something and had escaped error.[2]

Perhaps the greatest example of the truth of Bernard's quote are the voyages of Christopher Columbus (1451–1506) to explore the path to Asia. Columbus believed that he could get to India by sailing west from Spain. He arrived in the Caribbean in 1492 and named the local people "Indians" because he thought that he had arrived in India. Columbus was wrong, of course, although his adventure was monumentally fertile for human exploration.

There are many other important examples of the value of error. In 1968, a scientist at the headquarters of the 3M Company in Minnesota named Spencer Silver was trying to develop a strong new adhesive. He failed. Instead of inventing a heavy-duty adhesive he developed one that weakly stuck to surfaces and did not bind well. It took several years for the company to realize the value of their product, which is now its most successful creation: Post-It Sticky Notes.

There are also many examples of drugs developed for one purpose which turned out to be valuable for something else entirely. Minoxidil was intended as a blood pressure drug for treatment of hypertension—it was repurposed for hair growth.

---

* This book is highly readable. It is available at low cost from Dover Books in an English translation.

Sildenafil was developed by Pfizer to increase blood flow to the coronary arteries and became the first male potency-enhancing agent.

If you think a patient has a certain diagnosis because of several findings that support your chosen diagnosis, but there are others that indicate that the diagnosis is incorrect, this could be because it is incorrect or because the reasons that suggest that is incorrect are wrong. It could also be, of course, that the patient has two, three, or more conditions and that Occam's razor is violated.

Pediatric neurologist David B. Clark taught me a clinical aspect of this approach to error. He said that in each case we could "throw out" one finding. That is, if we believed a patient had a certain diagnosis and there was evidence against that diagnosis, we should not assume that the diagnosis must be wrong. This did not mean that the finding that did not fit our reasoning should be neglected, but that it should not be allowed to cancel other evidence.

Imagine that you are a graduate student in a large successful laboratory. The laboratory is devoted to disease A using method B. In a lab meeting, you have a suggestion that, based on some new evidence, method C may help in understanding the results of method B. There may be evidence to suggest that method C will not help. It's worth considering the possibility that this contradictory evidence is misleading. Hopefully you will be able to make the suggestion without fear of being criticized for being wrong.

Clinical and scientific discussions should be open to novel concepts. In the history of science, most new ideas are not immediately accepted. This is shown many times in the lessons in this book. When, in 1632, Galileo promoted the theory of Copernicus that the Earth revolved around the Sun he was not congratulated on this great discovery. The bottom line is it is likely that any really good idea will have evidence showing that it is an error. See also "No single theory ever agrees with all the facts in it domain" (Lesson 80).

One woman's noise is another woman's signal.
—Sir Bernard Katz 1979 (adapted)

If you shut your door to all errors truth will be shut out.
—Rabindranath Tagore[3]

References

1. Bernard C. *An Introduction to the Study of Experimental Medicine*. Dover Books; 1927.
2. Perutz M. *Is Science Necessary?* EP Dutton;1989: 194.
3. Tagore R. *Stray Birds*. Macmillan; 1917.

Lesson 48
Much of What We Know Is Wrong (So Don't Believe Everything You Read)

When I was in medical school, I was told that about half of what I was going to learn would turn out to be wrong. I didn't believe it—I thought that science had advanced so far that now my learning would be filled with facts, facts, facts, and more facts. I was wrong, and the reality is that much of what we believe today will also turn out to be wrong.

A 2016 review, "The natural selection of bad science," reports that "many prominent researchers believe that as much as half of the scientific literature—not only in medicine, but also in psychology and other fields—may be wrong."[1] This problem is increasing because of the expansion of predatory journals and the incentives for academic success. A 2013 paper in *Nature* concluded that about 3% of biology and medicine papers show textual similarities to papers produced by paper mills (businesses that sell false work and authorship to researchers who require publications for their career).[2]

I was taught that every neuron has only one neurotransmitter—wrong. I was also taught that in the adult brain no new neurons are produced—wrong. Furthermore, I was taught that the DNA of every species is unique and could not possibly be moved from one creature to another—wrong. I was taught as well that bacteria could not live in the stomach because of its acidic environment. Oh, that's also wrong. In the 1970s, it was believed that Parkinson's did not influence cognition and did not have a genetic component. Both of these ideas have been shown to be in error.

Barry Marshall is an Australian physician who suspected that bacteria in the stomach were the cause of peptic ulcer and gastric cancer. With his colleague, Robin Warren, he suffered academically and professionally because of this idea, which did not conform to the view prevalent at the time that bacteria could not live in the stomach because of its acid environment. Marshall and Warren were able to culture bacteria from stomach specimens because of a fortuitous error in the laboratory. Their 1983 paper showing the presence of the bacterium *Helicobacter pylori* in persons with peptic ulcer was initially rejected for publication. Attempts to infect animals were not successful. In 1984, Marshall demonstrated that by drinking the bacteria he was able to induce massive inflammation (gastritis) in his own stomach. He was able to subsequently cure his infection with antibiotics. In 2005, the Karolinska Institute in Stockholm awarded Marshall and Warren the Nobel Prize in Physiology or Medicine "for their discovery of the bacterium *Helicobacter pylori* and its role in gastritis and peptic ulcer disease." Marshall's Nobel Lecture is worth reading.[3]

Awareness that our knowledge is always incomplete is an important step in productive reasoning.

> The greatest obstacle to discovery is not ignorance; it is the illusion of knowledge.
> —Daniel Boorstin, American historian (adapted)[4]

> It's what we know already that often prevents us from learning.
> —Claude Bernard

References

1. Smaldino PE, McElreath R. 2016 The natural selection of bad science. *R Soc Open Sci.* 160384. http://dx.doi.org/10.1098/rsos.160384.
2. Van Norden R. How big is science's fake-paper problem? *Nature.* 2013 Nov 6;623(7987):466–7. doi:10.1038/d41586-023-03464-x.
3. Nobel Prize Organization. Barry Marshall Nobel lecture. 2005. https://www.nobelprize.org/prizes/medicine/2005/marshall/lecture/.
4. Boorstin DJ. *The Discoverers*. Penguin Random House; 1983.

Lesson 49
Smart People Make Mistakes

It is advisable for students to examine their teacher's feet before they decide that their teaching is faultless. If they do so, they will learn that their leaders have feet of clay. Despite your teacher's prominence they are all capable of error. Here are several examples of this important consideration. These examples demonstrate that these faults are not rare events of the past. Several examples are shown to emphasize the point that **no one is immune from error**.

On June 22, 1893, the British Naval Commander in the Mediterranean, Vice Admiral George Tryon, decided to take personal command of summer naval maneuvers. He ordered an about-face of two parallel rows of battleships. His officers pointed out that there would be a collision. A relatively simple calculation demonstrated that the combined turning circles of the ships was greater than the distance between them. Despite the danger the Vice Admiral did not change his order and his flagship *Victoria* was rammed by the battleship HMS *Camperdown*. Tryon refused to believe that the damage was serious and ordered the nearby vessels not to send their lifeboats. The *Victoria* sank, taking him and 350 sailors with it. It is reported that his last words were "It is all my fault." He was believed to be an excellent officer but a domineering personality.

There is a neurosurgeon in the United States who has operated on the wrong side of a patient's head, twice. On one occasion the patient, who had a brain tumor, was being prepared for surgery on the operating table when the surgeon asked to see the MRI films. Unfortunately, the images that were viewed were from a different patient who also had a brain tumor and had a very similar name to the patient on the operating table.

Tragically, Jessica Santillan, a 17-year-old patient at Duke University, died in 2003 after receiving a heart transplant because the donor was of a different blood type.[1]

In 2004, a NASA mission to Mars crashed into the planet because the parachute switches were installed upside down, causing the capsule to crash into the planet. The impact destroyed the 3-year, $264 million mission. An earlier ship sent to Mars by NASA also crashed (1999) because a command for thrust was sent using the wrong units (Imperial instead of metric).

A research volunteer died in the 1990s in a study of methionine metabolism at Case Western Reserve University in Cleveland. The research participant received a substantial overdose of the amino acid methionine because the worker who prepared it for administration did not understand the meaning of a decimal point.[2]

On August 10, 1628, the Swedish warship *Vasa* was launched after a rushed building program. Sweden was at war with Poland at the time, and King Gustavus Adolphus desperately wanted more warships for his campaign. It is recorded that the king requested that more cannons be put on the top level of the ship to make it more frightening to the enemy. (The ship had 64 bronze cannons.) The ship's designer could not be consulted about this because he had died a year before the ship was launched. Before sendoff the ship was tested and found to be unstable. Nonetheless, when it was launched it sailed into the Stockholm Harbor and sank after traveling 1,300 meters, when a light wind caused it to keel over on its side, with water rushing into the gun portals. Clearly the ship was top-heavy, which contributed to its instability. The sinking was a blow to the king's war efforts, and 53 sailors died in the disaster.[3] Apparently no one had the courage to question the tragic order of the king to move the cannons up to the top level.

Galileo Galilei was a brilliant Italian engineer, astronomer, and physicist. He was aware of the theory of Johannes Kepler that the tides were caused by the gravitational attraction of the moon. He preferred his idea, that the rotation of the earth was a better explanation. He was famously wrong.

An incident known as the Ferry Catastrophe involved a ship coming from Stockholm to Tallin in Estonia. The ferry sank in the Baltic Sea, killing 852 people on September 28, 1994. It sank because the door through which the cars drove into the bottom of the ferry had not been properly closed. You don't need to know anything about naval architecture to know that if a giant ferry door is not sealed properly, disaster will occur. Thus, the problem was obvious, simple, and tragic.

The Deepwater Horizon was an ultra-deep-water semi-submersible offshore drilling oil rig which experienced a blowout and explosion on April 20, 2010, which killed 11 workers and injured 17. The rig was celebrated for its advanced design and was one of the most powerful in the world, an industry model for safety. The oil spill which resulted from the explosion released 210 million gallons of crude oil into the Gulf of Mexico for 87 days, making it the largest oil spill in US history and the nation's second largest manmade environmental disaster. Investigations concluded that the tragedy was the result of poor risk management, failure to respond to critical indicators, and inadequate response training.[4] The workers were concerned that they would be fired for raising safety concerns and turned off operational alarms because they interfered with sleep.[5]

Albert Einstein was also noted to have made several surprising errors. Most notably, he refused to accept quantum mechanics as a fundamental theory.[6]

The great Rudolph Virchow, founder of cellular pathology, failed to appreciate the importance of the germ theory of disease developed by Louis Pasteur and the related demonstration of the importance of antisepsis by Ignaz Semmelweis (Lesson 34).

The general principle concerning the conclusion that "smart people make mistakes" is that **there is no error that is so obvious, so critical, and so deadly that it cannot be made. And no person is so prominent, famous, brilliant, and well-respected that** they are not capable of making a horrible mistake. It is vital to maintain awareness of this reality.

The reasons why I have emphasized the importance of recognizing error are (1) your imagination is enhanced by understanding that everything you know may not be correct and (2) making mistakes is an integral part of science, and recognizing that you are wrong can be an important step toward progress.

> A kernel of truth sticks in every error.
> —Rudolph Virchow[7]

References

1. Editorial. A death at Duke. *N Eng J Med*. 2003;348:1083–4.
2. Cottington EM, LaMantia C, Stabler SP, Allen RH, Tangerman A, Wagner C, Zeisel SH, Mudd SH. Adverse event associated with methionine loading test: A case report. *Arterioscler Thromb Vasc Biol*. 2002 Jun 1;22(6):1046–50. doi:10.1161/01.atv.0000020400.25088.a7. PMID: 12067919.
3. Fairley RE. Why the Vasa sank: 10 lessons learned. https://faculty.up.edu/lulay/failure/vasacasestudy.pdf
4. Broder JM. BP shortcuts led to Gulf oil spill, report says. *New York Times*. Sep 14, 2011.
5. Rothenberg DH. *Situation Management for Process Control: Situation Awareness and Decision Making for Operators in Industrial Control Rooms and Operation Centers*. International Society of Automation (ISA); 2019.
6. Krauss L. What Einstein got wrong: Everyone makes mistakes. But those of the legendary physicist are particularly illuminating. *Sci American*. 2015.
7. Virchow R. *Disease, Life and Man*. Stanford Studies in the Medical Sciences IX; 1938.

Lesson 50
Fishing Expeditions May Be Productive

There is widespread criticism of investigations that appear to lack sufficient justification. This critique can be applied to diagnostic testing as well as scientific investigations. At times the criticism of a project as being a "fishing expedition" can certainly be valid. For example, an electroencephalogram (EEG) is not indicated for every patient with headache. However, there are times when questions can be pursued without specific hypotheses. Space travel is a good example. Certainly, the first views of the far side of the moon by Soviet probe Luna 3, in 1959, was a valid endeavor not requiring a hypothesis. When a new tool becomes available it is often fruitfully and widely applied without specific predetermined ideas.

Parkinson's disease has no known cause in the 90% of cases that are not caused by a genetic anomaly. It has been learned only in the past 10 years that significant abnormalities in the gut may be the initiating site of the pathological process of the disease. German American neurologist Frederick Lewy first described the brain pathology of the disease in 1912.[1] Why did it take about a hundred years to discover that there were also important changes in the intestines in Parkinson's? Certainly, a proposal to investigate all the body systems in Parkinson's 40 years ago would have been criticized as a fishing expedition. If properly carried out it might have significantly expedited our understanding of the disease.

In 2021, NASA reported that the first flight of their Mars helicopter stirred up dust clouds which might help them to understand natural dust storms on the planet. Planetary scientists determined that dust could be transported in the thin air of Mars more easily than they had suspected. Planetary scientist Jim Bell said "there's an unanticipated atmospheric science experiment coming out of this." The goal of the mission was only to see if the helicopter could fly. Plans for the observations of the effect of the helicopter on the Martian surface could have been criticized as a fishing expedition (perhaps especially foolish for a planet without fish). But, fortunately, the scientists were open to see what happened. Physicist Brian Jackson said, "anything we can learn from it scientifically is icing on the cake." We should all be open to the possibilities of icing on cakes as we learn from our powers of observation.[2]

Neurologist Robert Joynt of the University of Rochester said that anyone who criticized a scientific project for being a fishing expedition had never been fishing. He explained that a person fishing goes out at a certain time, equipped with specific tools, and proceeds with specific procedures allowing for a successful outing.

If we require every clinical or scientific endeavor to have a well-developed hypothesis, we will impair our ability to use our powers of observation to make advances.

Frederick Lewy (1885–1950): A Person to Know

Lewy was a German American neurologist and the discoverer of Lewy bodies, a chief pathology of Parkinson's disease and Lewy body dementia, a condition named after him.[1] Because of the rise of Nazism in Germany he was forced as a Jew to emigrate to London and then to Philadelphia, where he served as Chief of Neurology at an Army hospital. He contributed important studies on peripheral nerve injuries, animal research, and the functions of the cerebellum. Most importantly, he expanded the localization of pathology in Parkinson's disease from the basal ganglia to the cortex[1] (see Lesson 67).

References

1. Holdorff B. Friedrich Heinrich Lewy (1885–1950) and his work. *J Hist Neurosci.* 2002 Mar;11(1):19–28. doi:10.1076/jhin.11.1.19.9106. PMID: 12012571.
2. Witze A. Mars helicopter kicks up "cool" dust clouds—and unexpected science. *Nature.* 2021 Jun 16;594(7864):484. doi:10.1038/d41586-021-01537-3. PMID: 34135498.

Lesson 51
Manifestations of Bias

> A bias is any predictable error that inclines your judgment in a particular direction.
> —New York Times

> A tendency, inclination, or leaning towards a particular characteristic, behaviour, etc.; a propensity. Also: something, especially an action or practice, to which a person is inclined or predisposed.
> —Oxford English Dictionary Online

Our evolutionary history has fostered the development of *bias* because it is adaptive for our preferences and fears to be influenced by our experiences. A woman I know was accidently locked in a room with chickens when she was 4 years old. The birds did not injure her, but one did sit on her shoulder. Since then, she has a fear of all birds and is unable to eat chicken.

Consider the tomato. The Solanaceae family of plants includes tomatoes and potatoes as well as deadly nightshade. Tomatoes originated in South America and were used in the sixteenth century in Italy as ornamental plants, and thought to be a form of deadly nightshade. They were believed to be toxic. A sixteenth-century book said that the tomato was "of ranke and stinking savour" and described the fruit as corrupt, with toxic leaves and stalk. The similarity of the two plants, deadly nightshade and tomatoes, led to a bias against consumption of tomatoes which lasted until the mid-1800s.

Many forms of bias can influence our judgment concerning medical and scientific problems. It is desirable, but not possible, to be completely free of all forms of bias. **The critical matter is to be aware of the potential for bias so that proper judgments can be made.** The author Arthur C. Clarke presented the reality that the forms of our biased reactions are powerful and that a completely open mind is not possible. He said, "One can only prepare for the unpredictable by trying to keep an open and unprejudiced mind—a feat which is extremely difficult to achieve, even with the best will in the world. Indeed, a completely open mind would be an empty one, and freedom from all prejudices and preconceptions is an untenable ideal."[1]

A list of different kinds of bias that are involved in medicine and science is presented below and in the next few lessons. This discussion of bias is not complete; review of all forms of bias would require a large book. Many of these forms of bias can be overlapping. That is, more than one form of bias can apply to a certain situation.

Another form of bias is the belief that you're not biased. This is a form of denial. Being smart does not mean you're not biased![2]

Bias against new ideas. This is certainly a common form of bias. Consider the introduction of the stethoscope by Rene Laennec. The *London Times* reported in 1834, "That it will ever come into general use notwithstanding its value ... is extremely doubtful: because its beneficial application requires much time and gives a good bit of trouble both to the patient and the practitioner; because its hue and character are foreign, and opposed to all our habits and associations.... There is something even ludicrous in the picture of a grave physician proudly listening through a long tube applied to the patient's thorax."[3]

Bias in favor of new ideas. There are physicians who always like to prescribe the latest drug that has been developed. There are also investigators who like to join the bandwagon of new scientific paradigms.

Framing bias: the way information is presented influences thought. This is a particularly potent and widespread form of bias. In the United States, the issue of abortion is presented as either "pro-life" or "pro-choice." Each side frames the matter in a way that favors their position, as we are all in favor of life and also all in favor of choice. If you have a patient who is a priest you may assume that he does not have a sexually transmitted disease because of the framing effect of liturgical clothing.

If you see a patient who tells you of a very strong family history of an inherited disease, you may be biased to believe that the patient has the condition which is running in his family. This may be an error, of course. If you are not aware of this bias, you may fail to consider nongenetic causes.

Overconfidence bias: from a false sense of talent or skill. In the 1990s, a brief tornado struck Cleveland, Ohio, and two people were killed. One was struck by a falling branch while sitting in his car. The other was a man who came upon a live wire that had fallen onto the street. It was reported that the wire was sparking as it jumped up and down on the wet pavement. The man stopped his car near the wire, got out, and yelled for everyone to stand back. He told the crowd that the wire was dangerous, that he was an electrician, and that he knew how to handle it. He walked up to the wire, picked it up, and was electrocuted.

Ueli Steck was one of the world's greatest mountaineers. He preferred to climb alone without any rope or other protection. This allowed him to set speed records for many climbs. He climbed on vertical ice and rock surfaces with only two ice axes and *crampons*, devices put onto shoes to help hold securely to ice and snow, and with no ropes. Climbing in this manner is extraordinarily hazardous. Even though he may have been the world's greatest mountain climber, he was still subject to the laws of gravity. He died of a fall of more than 1,000 meters at age 40, in 2017, while training on Nuptse, a 7,861-meter peak 2 kilometers away from Everest in Nepal.

Availability bias explains our likelihood to judge an event by our most common experience. The French call this *déformation professionelle*, the tendency to look at everything from the perspective of one's profession.[4]

Confirmation bias occurs when you observe only those features that you expect and neglect those you do not expect, thus confirming your erroneous judgment before you have completed your evaluation.[5]

Desirability bias occurs when you see what you want to see. Confirmation and desirability bias may occur because of a lack of indifference. In a one-page essay, "The importance of indifference in scientific research," biophysicist Martin Schwartz suggests we consider a policy of "passionate disinterest."[6] Since science is a conversation with nature it is best that our preconceived ideas do not alter our analysis. He suggests we practice nonattachment.

Attribution errors attributes phenomena to something other than their real cause. This may involve attributing your success to your great skill and attributing failure to factors beyond your control. **Self-serving bias** may be a form of attribution bias. Results supporting an hypothesis are accepted as valid and widely publicized. Results which do not support an hypothesis are considered to represent an error, which does not require publication.

Diagnosis momentum can occur when these forms of bias lead to an incorrect diagnosis being maintained through time with varying doctors despite evidence suggesting that it is erroneous. I saw a patient in a Veterans Administration hospital who had been seen for more than 20 years with the diagnosis of multiple sclerosis (MS). The diagnosis had been made based on his abnormal eye movements. In my examination, I noted that his oculomotor abnormality was pendular nystagmus, in which the direction of jerking of each eye was the same, like that of a pendulum. This indicated he had a congenital abnormality unrelated to MS. The erroneous diagnosis had been carried on through more than 20 years of neurology clinic visits. All the other physicians he had encountered in the past 25 years failed to recognize the erroneous diagnosis because of diagnosis momentum (a form of **anchoring bias**).

Commission bias occurs when the impulse is to be active rather than passive. This can be caused by a failure to appreciate that the data are not suitable to suggest a course of action. There are times, of course, when the best thing to do is to do nothing.[5] This may be noted at the time of end of life when no viable treatments are available, yet clinicians continue with therapies that are not enhancing the patient's quality of life.

Herd mentality: in-group bias, copying others. This form of bias is extensive in science and medicine and is often referred to as "jumping on the bandwagon." In the 1950s and 1960s, it was widely recommended that milk and cream were effective for peptic ulcer. There were no data to support this recommendation, and later studies showed that dairy products had a negative effect on peptic ulcers.

Narrative fallacy: The tendency to invent a story explaining something that happened based on random features.[7] In our attempt to make sense of the world, we may decide that two events that happen close to the same time must be related when there may actually be no relationship. Statistician Naseem Talib supports the view that we often make more cause-and-effect relationships than can it be supported by reality in his book *Fooled by Randomness*.[8]

Anchoring bias: This is the tendency to use preexisting data to judge future data. We often depend heavily on the first piece of information we receive (the anchoring fact). This form of bias is widespread and is actually close to the way science works. We use preexisting data to frame our understanding of new data. If you are asked to see a patient and told that the patient has a certain condition, you will be biased to believe that the anchoring fact (the diagnosis you were given for the patient) was correct. As with all forms of bias, it is critical to be aware that your study of a patient will be influenced by your preconceived ideas.

Here is an example of anchoring bias. In 1956, Tina Negus, a teenage girl, was exploring Charlwood Forest in Leicester, in the United Kingdom. She found a rock with an unusual pattern suggestive of ferns, which she thought was a fossil. She brought the rock to the attention of the authorities who said that it was not a fossil because the rock was from an early stage of earth's history when there were no life forms. The museum professionals who analyzed the rock did not consider its unique features and were not open to discovery since they could not go beyond the anchoring bias which said that there could not be any fossils in that area. Later the rock was observed again by 16-year-old Roger Mason who brought it to geologists; they found it to be one of the most significant fossils ever discovered because it validated Darwin's theory of evolution by natural selection by demonstrating the existence of life in that early period (Precambrian). It is so old that it is not a plant or an animal. **It is critical to not limit your observations and analysis by your preconceived ideas** (or anyone else's preconceived ideas!). Of course, that is what we all do all the time. What is important is to be aware of it. An article about the discovery of the fossil is entitled "*Charnia masoni*, a fossil discovery that proves the importance of the social aspect of knowledge."[9],[*]

Confirmation bias: People like concepts that confirm to their preconceived ideas. This bias has us avoid data that doesn't fit our predetermined notions. It is not uncommon that research studies that fail to support the investigator's preconceived ideas are not published. This can be because a suitable journal cannot be found to publish a negative study or because the authors do not submit the work for publication. On the other hand, researchers are eager to support work that validates their preconceived ideas. This can lead to premature publication of incomplete results.

> What people should realize is that it takes some kind of iron censor within oneself not to fall too much in love with one's own theories.
>
> —Sydney Brenner[10]

Hindsight bias: This is the "we knew it all along" effect. In this form of bias, a person believes they have predicted an event before it occurred. A hiker went for a walk in the woods and came upon a clearing with a large barn. On one side of the barn, he

---

[*] The fossil was named after Roger Mason, who became a geologist.

noticed 10 targets and at the center of each target was an arrow. He saw that 50 meters away there was a man holding a bow and arrow looking very proud of himself. The hiker asked the archer, "That's incredible, how could you possibly get the arrow in the center of every one of these targets from this distance?" The archer replied, "No problem. First, I shoot the arrows, then I draw the targets."

Optimism bias: We are more likely to predict good outcomes than bad outcomes. This form of bias can lead to inaccurate prognostication (predicting what will happen in the future), especially when it occurs with denial.

Affinity bias: This is a positive bias for people with whom we share life factors. It is not surprising that physicians may identify with some patients more than others because of ethnicity, religion, education, or occupation. Physicians do not want any of their patients to be ill. However, the doctor's psychological response to the patient's illness may be more marked in patients who are more like the doctor. This form of bias may influence management. For example, a physician who is caring for a physician patient may order more tests than she would have for a non-physician patient because of the desire to impress the patient with a thorough evaluation. This can lead to unnecessary expenses and, at times, complications.[11] This form of bias should not be allowed to influence decisions or recommendations.

Sampling bias: Many observations are based on a nonrandom sampling of the intended population. A physician may note that a certain condition is becoming more common. This may be because it is becoming more common, or perhaps only because another practitioner for the condition has retired, leaving more patients for others. A study of smoking and Alzheimer's disease compared cases at a Veterans Administration hospital with community controls and found that smoking was more common in Alzheimer cases. It is likely that the results were biased by the fact that veterans have a higher prevalence of smoking than do nonveteran community members.[12]

Another form of sampling bias was demonstrated in a 1991 report that showed that the proportion of left handers in the population decreases with age (13% in 20-year old's, less than 1% in 80-year old's). It was also found that the chance that a left-handed Major League Baseball player would die in a given year was 1–2% higher than the chance that a right-hander would die. It was concluded that left-handers are at greater risk of death at any given age. It was speculated that left-handedness "may indicate covert neuropathological features" and increased susceptibility to accidents.[13]

The precise explanation of the relationship between left-handedness and mortality was disclosed 2 years later.[14] Persons who die at a relatively advanced age are more likely than persons who die at a younger age to have been exposed to a bias against left-handedness. Remember that the word "sinister" in Latin means "left," and children who were born left-handed were commonly forced to become right-handed. Thus, persons who are identified as right-handed who died at an advanced age are more likely than those who died at a young age to have been originally left-handed and forced to be right-handed. This analysis, as well as recent epidemiological studies, shows that left-handedness is not associated with an elevated risk of death.

Bias in favor of common conditions: It is easier to recognize things we have seen many times than it is to recognize things which we have not seen or have not seen recently or have not seen often. This is a reflection of how the nervous system works: repetition enhances memory. This bias can be best handled with the awareness that if you see a lot of disease A you may have difficulty recognizing different conditions which resemble disease A.

Bias in favor of rare conditions: Clinicians may also make errors in diagnosis if they misjudge features of the patient in order to make a diagnosis of a rare condition. This may happen because the clinician is specializing in the rare condition or if the clinician wants to show her expertise in making a difficult diagnosis.

A senior professor of mine had written a paper on a rare neurological complication of cancer and frequently made the diagnosis in error. The condition he had published is uncommon, and, by making the diagnosis, he gave himself an opportunity to discuss a paper he had written.

During my oral examination for certification by the American Board of Psychiatry and Neurology I was asked to examine a patient with severely slurred speech, nystagmus (jerking eye movements), tremor, and ataxia. I was being evaluated by three senior neurologists, had only 30 minutes, and could not understand the patient's speech. I tried to obtain a history through head nodding. Somehow, I reached the diagnosis of Holmes spinocerebellar ataxia. The three senior neurologists who were examining me asked me many questions concerning what I had observed and my conclusion. I could tell from the questioning that I had missed the diagnosis. After 30 minutes one examiner said "We are running out of time. Do you think the patient may have MS?" I immediately said, "Yes, yes, that's it of course, why didn't I think of that!?" Then I explained why MS was more likely than my suggested diagnosis. The problem was that I was mistakenly trying to show the examiners that I could make a brilliant diagnosis when all they wanted was for me to demonstrate my competence (I passed). My bias made me look for rare, and not common, conditions.

Bias of no clinical experience: Some physicians have little experience taking care of patients. They may be very experienced and knowledgeable about their specialty but their knowledge should not be confused with clinical experience. Radiologists and pathologists provide valuable insight into the practice of medicine and their input is often of great value. But we must remember that their knowledge is about the radiological procedure or pathological findings and not about how the patient does with a certain treatment or other management decision.

In 2010, I was appointed to the Kentucky Spinal Cord and Head Injury Research Board. I learned about the animal model of spinal cord injury that was used. I suggested that the Board consider studies of what I consider to be a more appropriate animal model, with trauma to the back of the anesthetized animal and not to the naked cord (Lesson 44). My proposal was not accepted. I learned that the review committee that determined the recipients of funding was composed entirely of PhDs and contained no MDs. The clinical experience which physicians have provides vital insights into the nature of disease that cannot be obtained from books. The board members may have been biased by the fact that they had not cared for patients and did not understood the importance of the accuracy of the animal model.

Implicit bias is that which is not communicated directly (Cambridge English Dictionary) and is composed of assumptions that you are not aware of. Implicit bias is automatic and unintentional. Unconscious assumptions may be based on gender, skin color, sexual orientation, or other aspects of appearance. Everyone has prejudices that affect their perceptions and judgments; some are aware of these prejudices, and many are not.[15] Studies show that doctors have an unconscious preference for White over Black patients and for certain sexual orientations or religions.[16] This bias can affect diagnosis and treatment and contribute to health disparities.

Research has shown that women of color with chest pain waited longer to be treated in the emergency room, compared with White men. Also, doctors tend to underestimate pain reported by women and people of color. These biases may be reflected in the body language observed during patient–physician interactions. Research also shows there is a relationship between the amount of bias and lower quality of care.

It is difficult to know how to reverse these biases that are the results of centuries of White supremacy. The first step is awareness, and, to this effect, training exercises for students, physicians, and residents are being developed. Physicians in Massachusetts are required since 2022 to take training in implicit bias to get a new license or to be recertified.[15]

Bias can be identified in an unfortunate episode in the history of immunology. Elie Mechnikoff (1845–1916) was a Moldavian zoologist who observed cells in starfish larvae that engulf and ingest debris, which he named *phagocytosis*.[17] This is the key step in innate immunity. Around the same time the German physiologist Emil von Behring (1854–1917) developed antitoxins for diphtheria and tetanus, now known as *antibodies*, which are the central feature of the adaptive immune response. Metchnikoff and Behring were so opposed to each other that they could not see how their work could be combined for a unified understanding of immunity (i.e., Metchnikoff's work was the origin of innate immunity and von Behring's efforts the beginning of adaptive immunity). Metchnikoff and Behring won the 1908 Nobel Prize in Physiology or Medicine together. Metchnikoff did not attend the prize ceremony, possibly because he did not want to see Behring being honored. The difficulty between Metchnikoff and von Behring may have been a combination of confirmation bias and desirability bias.

Several other forms of bias are of interest. Racial bias as well as gender bias have received increasing attention in the past few years. The reader is referred to these works by Kahn[18] and Ross[19] for further discussion of these forms of bias.

Several of these forms of bias can act together. Consider the tragedy of frontal lobotomy.[20] This barbaric and tragic procedure procedure was developed by psychiatrist Walter Freeman, who thought that since mental illness was a product of abnormally functioning frontal lobes, disconnection from that part of the brain would relieve mental symptoms. The procedure was supported by prominent psychiatrist Adolph Meyer, president of the American Psychiatric Association and coiner of the term "mental hygiene." Another dangerous approach to mental illness supported by Meyer was the focal toxin theory that bacteria and rotting teeth caused mental illness. This led to tooth extraction and colonic resection as treatments for mental illnesses. Unfortunately, the fact that these radical measures did not work and had serious negative effects did not stop them being used in thousands of cases.[20]

It is likely that the widespread use of frontal lobotomy was an example of herd mentality ("jumping on the bandwagon"). Adolph Meyer was a powerful force in psychiatry at the time. Also, António Egas Moniz (1874–1955) received the 1949 Nobel Prize in Physiology or Medicine "for his discovery of the therapeutic value of leucotomy in certain psychoses." (Leucotomy is severing white matter tracts in the brain.) It remains one of the most controversial Nobel Prizes ever awarded.

Elie Mechnikoff (1845–1916): A Person to Know

Mechnikoff was a Russian zoologist and cofounder of the field of immunology. He observed cells moving in the body of starfish larva and from this developed the theory of phagocytosis. "Our wandering cells, the white cells of our blood—they must be what protects us from invading germs." He was a close associate of Louis Pasteur and believed that declines in aging were due to the toxic products of bacteria in the gut.

Emil von Behring (1854–1917): A Person to Know

Von Behring was a German physiologist and winner of the first Nobel Prize in Physiology or Medicine (1901) for the development of a therapy for diphtheria and tetanus based on serum antitoxin. Working as an assistant to Robert Koch in Berlin, he developed the serum therapy using sheep and horses in work with Paul Ehrlich. The therapy saved the lives of thousands of children and adults. Behring claimed the financial benefits of the work for himself and mistreated Ehrlich.

Paul Ehrlich (1854–1914): A Person to Know

Ehrlich was a German physician and scientist and winner of the 1908 Nobel Prize in Physiology or Medicine (together with Elie Metchnikoff). He contributed to treatments for syphilis and introduced the concept of chemotherapy (the magic bullet, an ideal therapeutic agent). Working under Robert Koch in Berlin, he developed, with Emil Behring, antitoxin therapy for the treatment of tetanus and diphtheria. He also discovered new ways to stain tissue to assist in the diagnosis of hematological disorders. He did not have good relations with either von Behring or Metchnikoff.

Robert Koch (1843–1910): A Person to Know

Koch was a German physician and scientist, and winner of the 1905 Nobel Prize in Physiology or Medicine for the identification of the bacteria that causes tuberculosis. He also studied tuberculin, a substance formed by the tuberculosis bacteria, which he erroneously believed could be used in the treatment of the disease. He also contributed to the bacterial understanding of anthrax and cholera, and, with Louis Pasteur, is considered a father of microbiology. He developed four principles to document the relationship between a pathogen and disease, referred to as *Koch's postulates*.[†]

> A great many people think they are thinking when they are merely rearranging their prejudices.
> —William James

> There is no way of telling where a particular line of research will lead.... And if you have [science] you cannot take only what you like. You have to accept as well the unexpected and disturbing results.
> —Francois Jacob, winner of the 1965 Nobel Prize in Physiology or Medicine

> It is necessary to be aware of the potential fallibility of all human actions.
> —Emil von Behring

References

1. Arthur C. Clarke: Use your imagination to see the future. December 2017. https://fabiusmaximus.com/2017/12/27/arthur-c-clarke-hazards-of-prophecy-lack-of-imagination/. Accessed 8/2024.
2. Grant A. *Think Again: The Power of Knowing What You Don't Know*. Viking; 2021.
3. Feinstein A. *Clinical Judgment*. Williams and Wilkins; 1967:390.
4. Horowitz A. *On Looking: A Walker's Guide to the Art of Observation*. Scribner; 2013.
5. Groopman J. *How Doctors Think*. Mariner Books; 2008: 179.
6. Schwartz MA. The importance of indifference in scientific research. *Company of Biologists*. 2016;128:2745–6.
7. Kahneman D. *Thinking, Fast and Slow*. Farrar, Straus and Giroux; 2013.
8. Talib N. *Fooled by Randomness: The Hidden Role of Chance in Life and in the Markets*. Incerto; 2005.
9. Vila J. Charnia masoni: A fossil discovery that proves the importance of the social aspect of knowledge medium. Aug 23, 2021. https://medium.com/thoughtsthatbyte/charnia-masoni-a-fossil-discovery-that-proves-the-importance-of-the-social-aspect-of-knowledge-525ae45db7c9.

[†] A movie series, *Charite*, presents a realistic recreation of the interactions of Koch, von Behring, and Ehrlich based in the hospital in which they worked.

10. Brenner S, as told to Louis Wolpert. *My Life in Science*. BMC Biomedcentral; 1994.
11. Hachinski V. Poets as guides in medicine, research, and life. *Neurology*. 2023 Oct 17;101(16):721-2. doi:10.1212/WNL.0000000000207582. Epub 2023 Jul 25. PMID: 37491323; PMCID: PMC10585671.
12. Shalat SL, Seltzer B, Pidcock C, Baker EL Jr. Risk factors for Alzheimer's disease: A case-control study. *Neurology*. 1987 Oct;37(10):1630-3. doi:10.1212/wnl.37.10.1630. PMID: 3658170.
13. Halpern DF, Coren S. Handedness and lifespan. *N Engl J Med*. 1991 Apr 4;324(14):998. doi:10.1056/NEJM199104043241418.
14. Salive ME, Guralnik JM, Glynn RJ. Left-handedness and mortality. *Am J Public Health*. 1993 Feb;83(2):265-7. doi:10.2105/ajph.83.2.265. PMID: 8427338; PMCID: PMC1694599.
15. Ortega RP. Do no unconscious harm. *Science*. 2023 Mar 3;379(6635):870-3. doi:10.1126/science.adh3698. Epub 2023 Mar 2. PMID: 36862779.
16. Weiner SJ, Schwarz A. *Listening for What Matters: Avoiding Contextual Errors in Health Care*. Oxford University Press: 2016.
17. Vikhanski L. *Immunity: How Elie Metchnikoff Changed the Course of Modern Medicine*. Chicago Review Press; 2016.
18. Kahn J. *Race on the Brain: What Implicit Bias Gets Wrong About the Struggle for Racial Justice*. Columbia University Press; 2018.
19. Ross HJ. *Everyday Bias: Identifying and Navigating Unconscious Judgments in Our Daily Lives*. Rowman and Littlefield; 2020.
20. Ghaemi SN. *The Rise and Fall of the Biopsychosocial Model* Johns Hopkins University Press; 2010.

Lesson 52
Experimenter Bias

Because of my bias in favor of the importance of experimenter bias, I have chosen to have this topic occupy an entire lesson.

Researchers can influence results in experimental work through their conscious and unconscious actions. For example, the researcher may have hypothesized that A caused B. When evaluating the results of the experiment she may, with or without awareness, alter the results so that the hypothesis is supported. It is difficult and perhaps impossible for people to be completely objective in making important observations.

In an elegant series of experiments, Rosenthal and colleagues demonstrated in 1964 that experimenter bias (also called *researcher bias*) can affect the results of a study of learning in rats.[1] Participants were asked to test the learning of rats they were given; some rats were reported to be slow learners and others noted to be smarter. Although the rats were genetically identical, it was found that the rodents identified as bright learned the tasks faster than those rats identified as dull. Because of this powerful source of bias in experimental work it is critical that observers be blinded whenever possible about which group their research participants may be in when conducting measurements.

When I was at the National Institute of Aging, I wanted to see if Alzheimer's disease was related to the amount of intracranial calcification. Calcium homeostasis is important in age-related brain diseases, and calcium deposition in the choroid plexus and pineal gland is often seen in healthy people. No one had studied the amount of calcium deposition in these structures in Alzheimer's disease. (Actually, the phenomenon is more correctly referred to as *mineralization*, because silicon is present as well as calcium and other minerals.) We collected CT scan films of patients and controls and subjectively assessed the amount of calcium deposits seen in the brain of the participants. I was concerned that we might be biased because we could see from the scan which patients had brain atrophy and which did not, which suggests group membership (Alzheimer patients often have brain atrophy). To prevent myself and the other examiners from seeing the cortex, I had assistants cover the cerebral cortex in the scans so that the examiners could only see the central regions where the calcifications occur. We found no relationship between calcification and disease status.[2]

Experimenter biases are important in clinical research. Imagine an investigator conducting a clinical trial to see if a new drug she has developed will help to treat a disease. If the results of the study are positive, it may be that she and her collaborators will get to write an important paper, obtain a large grant, acquire promotion, and possibly create a new company and become wealthy. Because of this powerful opportunity of bias, studies need to be done in a double-blind manner whenever possible, in which both the participants and the investigators are unaware of which patient is receiving which experimental agent or procedure.

There are many opportunities for experimental bias to be involved in clinical trials. This is discussed in Lesson 52.

> For what a man had rather were true he more readily believes. Therefore he rejects difficult things from impatience of research; sober things, because they narrow hope; the deeper things of nature, from superstition; the light of experience, from arrogance and pride, lest his mind should seem to be occupied with things mean and transitory; things not commonly believed, out of deference to the opinion of the vulgar. Numberless in short are the ways, and sometimes imperceptible, in which the affections colour and infect the understanding.
> —Francis Bacon[3]

Francis Bacon (1561–1626): A Person to Know

Bacon was an English philosopher and a politician who promoted the scientific method and enhanced the development of the Scientific Revolution. He was a supporter of empiricism and rejected the philosophy of Aristotle, supporting the importance of observation of events rather than analysis of ideas. He promoted the value of scientific experimentation as a way to worship God. He served as legal counsel to Queen Elizabeth I and was an opponent of religious discrimination.

References

1. Rosenthal RR, Lawson R. A longitudinal study of the effect of experimenter bias on the operant learning of laboratory rats. *J Psychiatr Res*. 1964 Jun;2:61–72. doi:10.1016/0022-3956(64)90003-2. PMID: 14177091.
2. Friedland RP, Luxenberg JS, Koss E. A quantitative study of intracranial calcification in dementia of the Alzheimer type. *Int Psychogeriatr*. 1990 Spring;2(1):36–43. PMID: 2101296.
3. Bacon F. *Novum Organum* (1620). CreateSpace Independent Publishing Platform; Sep 11, 2017.

Lesson 53
Bias of the Lost Actors

This form of bias could also be referred to as "dead men tell no tales" (also known as *survivorship bias*[1]). We all have inaccurate ideas about reality because the information we have about the world comes only from the living. For example, I have read many books about mountaineering expeditions. They are all written by those who survive and show what a great time everyone had. Sir Edmund Hillary famously said of Everest: "Well, we knocked the bastard off!" It is not uncommon to read a story of a mountaineering "conquest" in which the trip is presented as a grand adventure, in which everyone had a great time—except for the person or persons who died.*

Bias of the lost actors applies as well to our clinical experience. If we think about the patients we have seen in clinic who had a certain condition and how they've done, we must realize that we only know about those who came back to see us. This form of bias is particularly potent in emergency medicine because many patients are seen by emergency room doctors only once.

This form of bias is also important in clinical trials. It is necessary to consider what happened to research participants who drop out of the study. Obviously, if all of the participants who had side effects drop out and the dropouts are not considered in the final results, the data about the effects of the agent tested will be inaccurate.

It is possible to confront this bias by searching out information about your patient's outcomes. For example, if you are on an emergency medicine rotation and you see a patient who goes to surgery the next day, it will be valuable for you to find out what happens to the patient. (Remember to be *fierce*; Lesson 4).

Reference

1. Miller B. How "survivorship bias" can cause you to make mistakes. BBC. Aug 28, 2020. https://www.bbc.com/worklife/article/20200827-how-survivorship-bias-can-cause-you-to-make-mistakes. Accessed Nov 2, 2023.

---

* I am fond of reading about mountaineering exploration because it is not dangerous. That is, no one has ever died reading about mountaineering.

Lesson 54
Being Smart Is Not Enough

Harvard psychologist Howard Gardner proposed a "theory of multiple intelligences," which proposes that the concept of intelligence as a unitary indicator of mental function is incomplete.[1] He outlined how there are important aspects of intellectual function other than memory, including visual-spatial aptitude, verbal skills, interpersonal awareness, mathematical capacities, and musical talents. Psychologist Daniel Goleman significantly expanded this idea by proposing the concept of *emotional intelligence*, which is related to social skills, empathy, motivation, self-awareness, and self-regulation.[2] (*Empathy* is the ability to understand and appreciate the feelings of another.) It is important to realize that there are cognitive capacities in all of us which are not well measured by intelligence testing.

In medicine and science, there is a long-standing tendency to treasure memory over all other cognitive functions. The theory of multiple intelligences and the importance of emotional intelligence illustrate the error of focusing on memory as a criterion of mental ability. Much of education measures only memory and not many other aspects of "intelligence." Widespread access to the internet makes memory talents less important than before. Focusing on memory abilities is misguided.

When I was a resident in neurology, we had a young attending physician who came from one of the major medical centers to work at Mount Sinai Hospital in New York. In one of his first hospital rounds in which he served as our attending, I presented a case to him. In the middle of the presentation, he said that he knew what the matter was with the patient and that it had been described in a recent paper in the journal *Neurology*. He then wanted to proceed to the next case. We asked him if he'd like to see the patient and he said that it would not be necessary. As far as this patient was concerned it didn't matter if the doctor was smart. What mattered was that he erroneously thought that he did not need to see the patient to determine what was going on. (This is an example of how hospital rounds should *not* be managed.)

If you know all the medical literature but are not a good observer, you are not a good doctor. If you know all the literature but you have poor judgment, you are not a good doctor. If you know all the literature but you are lacking in compassion, you are not a good doctor.

We all know that we can improve our memory, math, linguistic, and visual spatial abilities with practice. This is also true about our capacity for compassion and emotional awareness.

Let someone say of a doctor that he really knows his physiology or anatomy.... These are not real compliments; but if you say he is an observer, a man who knows how to see, this is perhaps the greatest compliment one can make.
—J. M. Charcot[3]

You can observe a lot by watching.
—Yogi Berra (1925–2015), American baseball player[4]

Jean-Martin Charcot (1825–1893): A Person to Know

Charcot, French neurologist and professor of pathology, is known as "the father of modern neurology." He played an important role in recognizing multiple sclerosis, amyotrophic lateral sclerosis (ALS; also known as motor neuron disease), and many other conditions. He also made important contributions in understanding functional neurological disorders, originally called hysteria. Charcot's teaching emphasized careful neurological examination and clinical-pathological correlation.

References

1. Gardner H. *Frames of Mind: The Theory of Multiple Intelligences*. Basic Books; 1994.
2. Goleman D. *Emotional Intelligence: Why It Can Matter More Than IQ*. Bantam Books; 1995.
3. Charcot E. *Oevres completes de JM Charcot*. A. Delahaye; 1988: 175.
4. Berra Y. *You Can Observe a Lot by Watching*. Turner Publishing; 2009.

Lesson 55
Don't Be Afraid of Your Imagination

It is well known that there are gut factors which cause the brain diseases kuru, scrapie, and bovine spongiform encephalopathy (BSE, mad cow disease). In 2015, I wondered if there could be gut factors responsible for Alzheimer's disease, Parkinson's disease, and amyotrophic lateral sclerosis (ALS) as well (99% of case of Alzheimer's and 90% of Parkinson's are not caused by genes). I learned that amyloid proteins are produced by bacteria, including organisms that reside in our intestines, such as *Escherichia coli*. In a hypothesis paper, I proposed that these bacterial products made by members of our microbiota (Gut microbes) caused the initiation of protein misfolding, which is a key mechanism of all three disorders.[1] I also hypothesized that these functional bacterial amyloid proteins primed the immune system, so it was more responsive to amyloid proteins developing in the brain with aging. Several friends ignored my ideas and one in England told me distinctly that I was a "nutter." My papers were challenging to get published.

The ideas I proposed have now been documented by my group and others, in studies of mice, nematodes (roundworms), and fruit flies (*Drosophila*), as well as work in vitro (taking place outside of an organism). The opportunity to prevent or treat this disease through medications targeting bacterial amyloid is being addressed in industry and labs in the United States, Israel, Denmark, Hong Kong, and Japan.[2]

The key factor responsible for this work is the question "What is responsible for initiating these diseases in those cases that are not inherited?" I did not allow my imagination to be limited by the fact that I'm not a protein biochemist and did not have a lab with 15 postdoctoral fellows and 10 graduate students. In retrospect, the key elements were respect for my imagination, openness to asking questions, and going beyond my neuroscientific silo.

The story of BSE also interesting questions which challenge our imagination. The epidemic of BSE in cows most likely resulted from the feeding of cows to cows. The development of cases in humans in Britain led to the appreciation that materials from cows can be infectious and can transmit the disease to both cows and humans. After the butchering of a cow is complete there is considerable material left over, which is used for animal feed and plant fertilizer (bone meal). This process is called *rendering*. In the 1990s, the use of rendered material from cows for feeding of cows was banned after the outbreak of BSE in which about 200 people died. How do you think the rendering industry responded to this ban?

In 2009, I learned that material from cows was being fed to fish in fish farms. The infectious agent of BSE, which is called a prion, is extraordinarily potent and resistant to inactivation. It is possible that a fish in a farm could act as a carrier and transmit the disease to a person eating the fish (fish were known to have a form of the prion protein). Robert Petersen and I proposed that the prion could infect the fish directly.[3] In our 2009 paper "Bovine spongiform encephalopathy and aquaculture," we proposed that the feeding of cows to fish should be banned because of the risk of transmission of the infectious agent.

Later that year it was demonstrated that BSE, and the prion disease of sheep called scrapie, can be transmitted to fish. Soon after I was called by the head of a rendering association, who asked me, "What can he do with all this material that cannot be fed to cows?" I suggested the best policy would be to burn it. I also discussed the matter with an official at the US Department of Agriculture about upcoming regulations about rendering. He concluded that the risk to human health was very small so that the feeding of rendered material from cows to fish would continue to be allowed.

I disagree with this conclusion. The risk may be maybe small, but it is not zero. I am sure that there are many people like me who eat fish but do not eat beef. We do not wish to be eating material from cows in our fish! Another matter is that the health benefits of fish are related, of course, to the nutritional value of the fish, which is related to the fish's diet. Fish in farms who are eating cows are not eating as much krill, insects, plankton, and other fish. The nutritional characteristics of the fish may be negatively affected. Nutritional differences between farmed and wild fish have been reported.[4] My summary of the matter is that fish do perfectly well in the sea without eating cows.[3]

Welcoming your own imagination is necessary for creativity. Be hospitable to your creativity—receive it warmly and make sure it feels at home in your mind. **Challenge conventional beliefs and respect your own wisdom.**

> It is a miracle that curiosity survives formal education.
>
> —Albert Einstein

References

1. Chen SG, Stribinskis V, Rane MJ, Demuth DR, Gozal E, Roberts AM, Jagadapillai R, Liu R, Choe K, Shivakumar B, Son F, Jin S, Kerber R, Adame A, Masliah E, Friedland RP. Exposure to the functional bacterial amyloid protein curli enhances alpha-synuclein aggregation in aged Fischer 344 Rats and Caenorhabditis elegans. *Sci Rep*. 2016 Oct 6;6:34477. doi:10.1038/srep34477. PMID: 27708338; PMCID: PMC5052651.
2. Wang C, Lau CY, Ma F, Zheng C. Genome-wide screen identifies curli amyloid fibril as a bacterial component promoting host neurodegeneration. *Proc Natl Acad Sci U S A*. 2021

Aug 24;118(34):e2106504118. doi:10.1073/pnas.2106504118. Erratum in: *Proc Natl Acad Sci U S A*. 2021 Oct 12;118(41): PMID: 34413194; PMCID: PMC8403922.
3. Friedland RP, Petersen RB, Rubenstein R. Bovine spongiform encephalopathy and aquaculture. *J Alzheimers Dis*. 2009;17(2):277–9. doi:10.3233/JAD-2009-1060. PMID: 19363268.
4. Modzelewska-Kapituła M, Pietrzak-Fiećko R, Kozłowski K, Szczepkowski M, Zakęś Z. Muscle tissue quality of raw and sous-vide cooked wild and farmed pikeperch. *Foods*. 2022 Nov 26;11(23):3811. doi:10.3390/foods11233811. PMID: 36496619; PMCID: PMC9735530.

Lesson 56
Do Not Assume That Your Ideas Are Not Novel and Important Just Because They Appear To Be Obvious

Nitrous oxide was first used as an anesthetic for the treatment of pain by the Boston dentist Horace Wells in 1844. He noted that a person who was intoxicated with the gas at a party fell and broke his leg but did not experience pain. He found the gas to be of value as an anesthetic in his dental practice. He was late in publishing his use of nitrous oxide because he assumed the value of the gas in dentistry was obvious to everyone. It wasn't.

Another idea which was rejected even though it is obvious is the use of cleanliness in the clinic and in the operating room and the need to wash your hands when leaving the morgue, as originally proposed by Ignaz Semmelweis and Joseph Lister[1,2] (Lesson 79).

Several times I have had ideas which appeared to be obvious to me. I would then go to the literature and learn that (1) my concepts are not novel and have already been thoroughly explored, (2) my idea is unlikely to be correct, or (3) perhaps no one had thought of it before. On one occasion I had an idea about a molecule involved in inflammation which I had never heard of before. I looked it up on the PubMed database and found more than 3,000 citations related to the molecule. On another occasion I had a thought about the interaction of two factors that could be involved in neurological disease. To my amazement, I found that apparently no one had worked on the idea before.

If you cannot find any previous work regarding an idea you have, it may be because (1) it's not a good idea; (2) it is a good idea, and other people are working on it but have not yet published about it; (3) other people have thought of the idea but haven't figured out how to test it; or (4) no one has thought of it before. Consider all possibilities.

In considering the potential value of your new idea, recognize that what is obvious to you may not be obvious to anyone else. Also, almost all great discoveries appear obvious in retrospect. If you are working in one field and have an idea that links that field to some other area, you may very well be the only person on earth who has thought that these two areas could be related in a specific manner.

> Science is made up of so many things that appear obvious after they are explained.
> —Frank Herbert, American science fiction author

References

1. Nuland S. *The Doctors' Plague: Germs, Childbed Fever, and the Strange Story of Ignac Semmelweis*. Norton; 2003.
2. Fitzharris L. *The Butchering Art: Joseph Lister's Quest to Transform the Grisly World of Victorian Medicine*. Farrar, Straus and Giroux; 2017.

Lesson 57
Consider the Evolutionary Aspects of Disease

Why does motion sickness cause nausea and vomiting? Why does food poisoning cause diarrhea? Why does systemic illness cause fatigue, fever, and malaise? Could these responses to illness have positive value? Evolution helps to answer these questions.

How could nausea be adaptive (enhance survival)? Nausea can be caused by the lack of proper balance between the vestibular system (balance) and vision. It is known that toxic exposures cause impairment of the complex interactions of balance and vision. The neurophysiology of the pyramidal tract (responsible for voluntary movement) is relatively simple, with two neurons from cortex to muscle. On the other hand, the interactions of the vestibular system and vision involve the semicircular canals, the eighth cranial nerves, several brainstem and cerebellar nuclei, and many connecting pathways. Thus, a 20% impairment in efficiency of the pyramidal tract may not cause noticeable loss of motor function but equivalent impairment in the interactions of balance and vision may produce impaired function. (Every time we turn our head our semicircular canals inform our eyes how to move to balance our visual world so that our sense of being stable is maintained.) This theory proposes that the intake of toxins that impair neurological function impair interactions of our visual and vestibular senses. Therefore, nausea may be adaptive, as a way to remove toxins from the body.[1]

Motion sickness is generally experienced when information from the ears does not agree with vision, thus mimicking the situation after toxin intake. The development of nausea and vomiting after food poisoning may also be appreciated as an evolutionary adaptive response to the intake of toxins.

You may recall how you feel when you had the flu or a bad cold. The feelings of fatigue and malaise as well as fever are not caused only by the infectious agents themselves. To a significant degree these responses are maintained by the body as an adaptive response helping us to rest. Interferons are proteins made by the body in response to viral exposure, and they inhibit viral replication. When they were first given to patients in the 1980s, it was found that interferons cause headache, malaise, and fever. 20,000 years ago, an ancestor of ours who had a throat infection would be more likely to do well if they rested as opposed to going out hunting and gathering. Thus, the feeling of malaise and fatigue with illness may be an adaptive response.

We like to eat sweets because they provide us with a rapid source of energy. Genetic features that enhance eating of sweets has not had a negative effect on survival because sugar was scarce for most of human history. Also, a genetic tendency to overeat sweets might actually be advantageous in a famine. Of course, the situation today is different.

Randolph Nesse is an American physician who is a founder of the field of evolutionary medicine and evolutionary psychiatry.[2] In a pivotal paper "What good is feeling bad: The evolutionary benefits of psychic pain,"[3] he asks why we are capable of depression and anxiety. He proposes that our experience of these emotions is adaptive because they signal the need for attention to what's happening in one's life and consideration of remediable actions.

The Austrian psychoanalyst Victor Frankel reported a patient of his who had been a patient of another analyst who had died.[4] The patient had been seeing another analyst for many years with multiple visits per week. The patient had been unhappy with his boss, but his first analyst had advised him not to resign his position until he could understand what the problem was with his relationship with his supervisor. At the second visit with Dr. Frankl, he was advised that if he didn't like his boss he should quit. He did so and reportedly his problem was removed. This illustrates the adaptive value of depression. To put it another way, Nesse points out that depression is not primarily caused by antidepressant deficiency.

As Nesse said, "Emotions are set to maximize Darwinian fitness, not happiness."[3] Bad feelings can be useful. For us to understand the forces behind depression and anxiety we need to learn about the patient. Psychopharmacology may help but it does not replace exploring the patient's life in its own context.

Evolutionary factors are involved in all our structural and functional features. I have often been asked how microbial features of the gut could affect the brain. My favorite answer is to explain that we all have more than 500 grams of live bacteria in the gut, which is comprised of perhaps 1 billion organisms, including 100 times more genetic information than that contained in our own DNA. This is our largest environmental exposure. Therefore, it is critical that our immune system be aware of what is happening with the microbiota (the bacteria, fungi, and other microbes that reside inside the digestive tract, including the mouth, nose, and intestines). In addition, it has been shown that the immune system influences gut microbiota in such a profound manner that the microbiota are "gardened" by the immune system (the immune system influences the population of organisms present). At the same time, the immune system is "educated" by the microbiota (the microbiota control the development of the immune system). If there were no opportunities for the immune system to know about what's happening in the gut, our ancestor's survival would have been threatened a very long time ago. Several pathways by which gut microbes can influence the brain have been described.[5]

A role for human evolution in the persistence of the apolipoprotein E e4 (Apo E e4) gene (allele) has been proposed. The E4 allele is highly associated with the risk of developing Alzheimer's disease. Why has it not been extinguished by evolution since it is associated with Alzheimer's, stroke, intracranial bleeding, and poor outcome after head injuries? We have reported that the malarial parasite does not grow as well in the blood of people who are e4 positive.[6] This suggests that a protective action of the gene may serve to enhance its representation in the population even though it has negative effects. This situation is called *antagonistic pleiotropy*, in which a gene that has a minor positive effect in early life will be favored even if its effects in later life are damaging.

You may ask why I keep bringing up evolution in a book on critical thinking. Evolution provides an important perspective on every aspect of brain function. The clearest view of the central nature of evolution is provided by Nobel laureate Sir John Eccles (1903-1997), "When we consider the story of the evolutionary development of living forms, we tend to regard ourselves as being onlookers at this evolutionary procession, as we try to hold in thought the immensity and wonderful productivity of this biological process. But we are *in* the procession. It is not enough for us to think of man in general as being so engaged. It is a sense of personal involvement that we must realize emotionally. Each of us, I and you, is at the end of a line of genetic descent that stems from the earliest living organisms."[7]

Viktor Frankl (1905-1997): A Person to Know

Frankl was an Austrian neuropsychiatrist and a founder of the logotherapy school of psychoanalysis. In 1942, he was sent to concentration camps in Poland, where his mother, father, and brother were murdered. His Holocaust experience was pivotal in developing the ideas expressed in his book *Man's Search for Meaning*, in which he teaches that people are free to decide how to respond to challenges and that the search for life's meaning was the most important motivational force.[4]

> Rather than assuming that negative feelings are symptoms of a physical abnormality or a dysfunctional personality, family or society, the therapist can consider the possibility that some suffering is part of a vital mechanism shaped by natural selection to help people survive in the environment.
> —Randolph Nesse[3]

References

1. Treisman M. Motion sickness: An evolutionary hypothesis. *Science*. 1977 Jul 29;197(4302):493-5. doi:10.1126/science.301659. PMID: 301659.
2. Williams GC, Nesse RM. The dawn of Darwinian medicine. *Q Rev Biol*. 1991 Mar;66(1):1-22. doi:10.1086/417048.
3. Nesse R. What good is feeling bad: The evolutionary benefits of psychic pain. *The Sciences*. Nov/Dec 1991:30-7.
4. Frankl V. *Man's Search for Meaning*. Beacon Press; 2006.

5. Friedland RP. *Unaging: The Four Factors That Impact How You Age*. Cambridge University Press; 2022.
6. Fujioka H, Phelix CF, Friedland RP, Zhu X, Perry EA, Castellani RJ, Perry G. Apolipoprotein E4 prevents growth of malaria at the intraerythrocyte stage: Implications for differences in racial susceptibility to Alzheimer's disease. *J Health Care Poor Underserved*. 2013 Nov;24(4 Suppl):70–8. doi:10.1353/hpu.2014.0009. PMID: 24241262; PMCID: PMC4909051.
7. Eccles J. Preface. In *The Human Mind*, a discussion at the Nobel conference, JD Roslansky, ed. North Holland Publishing; 1967: 3.

SECTION V
PERSONAL AND CAREER DEVELOPMENT

Lesson 58
Live in "Day-Tight Compartments"

The past is gone and will not return. The future has not yet arrived. The only choice left for us is to deal with the present. If your mind is engaged in regret and reimagining of past events, it is difficult to focus on the patient who is with you in the present moment. If your mind is focused on future expectations, anticipations, and fears, it is difficult to focus on the patient who is with you in the present moment. Learning is enhanced when your attention is not divided between the past and the future.

Awareness of the importance of the present moment was understood by the great Canadian American physician William Osler, who advised his students to live in "day-tight compartments."[1]

> As a patient with double vision from some transient unequal action of the muscles of the eye finds magical relief from well-adjusted glasses, so, returning to the clear binocular vision of to-day, the over anxious student finds peace when he looks neither back ward to the past nor forward to the future.... Now each one of you is a much more marvelous organization than the great liner (the Titanic), and bound on a longer voyage. What I urge is that you so learn to control the machinery as to live with "day-tight compartments"; as the most certain way to ensure safety on the voyage. Get on the bridge and see that at least the great bulkheads are in working order. Touch a button and hear, at every level of your life, the iron doors shutting out the Past—the dead yesterdays. Touch another and shut off, with a metal curtain, the Future—the unborn to-morrows. Then you are safe—safe for to-day!
>
> —William Osler[2]

The focus on the present moment is a central feature of Buddhism. Many of us experience the world through worries about the past and anxiety about the future without awareness of the present moment. The reality is that the past is gone and that the future has not yet arrived. If you are in a dentist's chair and preparing for a difficult root canal and the dentist approaches you with a large needle you can understandably feel anxious about the present moment. However, most of the experience of anxiety is in regard to what has happened or what is anticipated. Paying attention to the present moment is a central feature of meditation and deep listening (Lesson 10).

The importance of attention to the unique gift of each day is illustrated by the poem "Days" by Philip Larkin.[3]

If you believe that feeling bad or worrying long enough will change a past or future event, then you are residing on another planet with a different reality system.
—William James

References

1. Osler W. A way of life and address to Yale students (1913). ReadaClassic.com. reprinting 2010
2. Hirshbein LD. William Osler and the fixed period: Conflicting medical and popular ideas about old age. *Arch Intern Med*. 2001 Sep 24;161(17):2074–8. doi:10.1001/archinte.161.17.2074. PMID 11570935.
3. Larkin P. "Days" In Collected Poems. Farrar Straus and Giroux; 2001.

Lesson 59
Learn How to Learn and Enhance Your Learning Capacity

Many of you reading this book are already academically accomplished. You have challenged your higher cognitive functions involving attention, memory, judgment, language, spatial reasoning, emotional intelligence, and executive functions (important for cognitive control of behavior, flexibility, planning, reasoning, and problem-solving). You have already learned a lot about how you learn. Awareness of your mechanisms and pathways of learning is critical. Our brains are different, and we do not all learn in the same way. You can maximize your learning by appreciating the unique features of your own cognitive capacities.

There are three components to memory: encoding, storage, and retrieval. *Encoding* is the process by which a concept or an event is registered in the brain. The memory must then be *stored* in a way which allows for it to be recovered at a later time. *Retrieval* is the process of recovering the memory from storage. Forgetting can happen with deficits in any of these three components of memory. If you park your car in a garage and do not pay attention to where it is parked, you may not remember its location because of a failure of encoding. A failure of storage may result if you categorize a memory incorrectly, which can make it harder to recall later. Retrieval failures commonly occur when you cannot recall a concept or an event even though you have no problem in recognizing it when given a choice. This is why we would all prefer an exam allowing us to choose between four possible answers compared to an exam which involves filling in a blank.

It is necessary to consider the importance of all three aspects of memory. Recall is aided by attention at the time of encoding. Psychologist Endel Tulving pointed out that retrieval cues (such as conceptual categories) aid our memory.[1] Forgetting can result if the receival cues are inadequate. Encoding is assisted by involving various sensory processes in the experience being remembered—it is easier to remember an experience with a patient which has visual, auditory, tactile, and perhaps even olfactory aspects than it is to remember a fact that you read in a book, which is entirely visual.

It may be risky to give recommendations to everyone because of the variability of learning styles. With this admitted limitation I do have some suggestions for your consideration.

- *Ask questions.* When should you stop asking questions? **Never stop asking questions.**
- *Always have a little book with you* for notes, as discussed in Lesson 4.
- *Avoid multitasking* whenever possible. Computers can do profound multitasking with enormous efficiency. Humans do not do multitasking well. Usually when we think we're multitasking we're actually shifting attention from one thing to another rapidly with a loss of effectiveness. Recognition of the inefficiency of multitasking is important for learning and patient care. Limit multitasking because of its negative effects on awareness, judgment, and wisdom.[*]
- *Read now*, don't pile up books to read one day. (Don't try to impress people by the pile of books you intend to read.)
- *When you don't know a new word look it up* right away, don't wait.
- *Study the history of medicine and science.* The giants of the past were humans just like us. Learning how they worked, how they thought, and how they experimented is of great value (and fun as well) Lesson 73).
- *Read and learn widely.* Do not bury yourself in one narrow silo without awareness of what other people are doing in other fields. At the same time, you do need to limit your reading to find the right balance between focus and diffusion (this is not easy and requires attention).
- *If you read something of interest in the literature and have a question* that the paper does not address, consider writing to the paper's senior author. You may get no response. Or your question may awaken interest, and a life-changing interaction may develop. It's worth a shot.
- *Remember that you do not need to know everything* (that's impossible, of course) (Lesson 85).
- *Whenever possible read the original literature.* It is common that researchers cite important historical papers without ever reading them. Frequently, the discussion of important works includes inaccuracies because no one has actually read the original contribution. Reading the original work may yield important insights about technology, data analysis, and scientific reasoning.
- *Do not abandon your outside interests.* The brain works best when it has time to rest. You may find that some of your best ideas come to you when you are not actively thinking about your work. Physical activity is good for the health of the brain, and exposure to the natural world is particularly valuable.[2, †]
- *Sleep is necessary for survival.* Lack of sleep can contribute to hypertension, heart disease, stroke, and various forms of dementia. You learn better if you rest and get good sleep.
- *Meditation also helps with relief from stress.*

---

[*] Multitasking is also a risk for traffic and pedestrian accidents.
[†] Remember that Roger Bannister, a British neurologist, was the first to run a mile in 4 minutes in 1954.

- *Relaxation is an important factor for your learning.* Reading scientific biographies and autobiographies can be of great value, as well as great enjoyment. *My Life in Science* by Nobel laureate Sydney Brenner is an excellent place to start.[3]
- *If you are a procrastinator learn to make procrastination work for you.* See "How to procrastinate and still get things done" by Stanford University philosopher John Perry.[4]
- On exams read all questions twice before answering.

Respect the Limits of Your Cognitive Processing Capacity

If your patient has a complete blood count, for example, it is not necessary to remember the exact value of each item, especially if the result is normal. If your patient has a chronic illness and has had several surgeries over the years, it may be worth remembering the month and year when each procedure was performed. But it is probably not relevant to remember the exact date for the operation.

Excessive cognitive load in medical care can be enormous, and cognitive overload can lead to medical errors and burnout. Many health data management systems do not properly consider the "human in the loop." Artificial intelligence (AI) will soon be helping us with patient evaluation and decision-making. It is important to learn how to use AI in a way that facilitates learning and enhances patient care.

> No man is really happy or safe without a hobby, and it makes precious little difference what the outside interests may be botany, beetles or butterflies, roses, tulips, irises; fishing mountaineering or antiquities anything will do so long as he straddles the hobby and rides it hard.
>
> —William Osler

Endel Tulving (1927–2023): A Person to Know

Endel Tulving was an Estonian/Canadian cognitive psychologist who showed that memory involves not only having the information available but also being able to retrieve it.[1] He disclosed the difference between various forms of memory, particularly semantic and episodic memory. *Episodic memory* is the recall of a personal experience (such as a visit to a car dealer) and *semantic memory* is the recall of information (general knowledge of the world, such as the information that Saab Automotive went defunct in 2011).‡ Tulving's work showed that episodic memory involves the

---

‡ The word "semantic" means related to meaning or significance.

medial temporal lobes of the brain, including the hippocampus. He postulated that the ability to move backward and forward in time is limited to humans.

Sydney Brenner (1927–2019): A Person to Know

One of the leading biologists of the twentieth century, Brenner was iconoclastic and superbly creative. He was so young when he graduated medical school that he was not able to practice medicine, so he turned to research. He was stimulated by the discovery of the DNA double helix by James Watson and Francis Crick in 1953. He made so many important discoveries in molecular biology that it was hard for the Nobel committee to decide which one merited his prize (2002). His work on the nematode *Caenorhabditis elegans* provided an unprecedented analysis of neural development. He was described as, "One of biology's mischievous children: the witty trickster who delights in stirring things up".[5]

References

1. Tulving E, Markowitsch HJ. Episodic and declarative memory: Role of the hippocampus. *Hippocampus.* 1998;8(3):198–204. doi:10.1002/(SICI)1098-1063(1998)8:3<198::AID-HIPO2>3.0.CO;2-G. PMID: 9662134.
2. Chen C, Nakagawa S. Physical activity for cognitive health promotion: An overview of the underlying neurobiological mechanisms. *Ageing Res Rev.* 2023 Apr;86;101868. doi:10.1016/j.arr.2023.101868. Epub 2023 Feb 2. PMID: 36736379.
3. Brenner S, as told to Louis Wolpert. *My Life in Science.* BMC Biomedcentral; 1994.
4. Perry J. How to procrastinate and still get things done. *Chronicle of Higher Education.* Feb 23, 1996. https://www.chronicle.com/article/how-to-procrastinate-and-still-get-things-done/.
5. Kenyon C. Sydney Brenner (1927–2019). *Science.* 2019 May 17;364(6441):638. doi: 10.1126/science.aax8563. PMID: 31097656.

Lesson 60
Find Out Where You Find Meaning

Consider the ideas of three Austrian psychiatrists. What did they believe was the primary human motivating force? The most well-known, Sigmund Freud (1856–1939), believed that it was sex (the pleasure principle). Alfred Adler (1870–1937), the Austrian psychotherapist and founder of the school of individual psychology, proposed that it was the will to power ("striving for superiority"). Viktor Frankl (1905–1997), the founder of the logotherapy school of psychoanalysis, believed that that it was man's search for meaning.[1]

Frankl was a victim of the Holocaust and survived imprisonment in Auschwitz. His experience as a doctor in the concentration camp taught him that survival was related to the ability of the victims to find meaning in their life. He said, "Those who have a 'why' to live can bear almost any 'how.'"[1] The search for meaning is an important individual process for all of us.

The choice of work activities is certainly an important step that requires careful thinking. No one can make such a choice for you. There are many ways in which you can find meaning in work and elsewhere. You may find meaning through healing, counseling, and contributing to science and healthcare, as well as to family. All young doctors and scientists must consider these questions carefully.

Victor Frankl's *Man's Search for Meaning* was written over a 9-day period following his release from Auschwitz and was published in 1946.[1] The English translation (1959) was an international bestseller. The US Library of Congress has named the book one of the 10 most influential books in the United States.

> The deepest principle in human nature is the craving to be appreciated.
> —William James

> To be sure, man's search for meaning may arouse inner tension rather than inner equilibrium. However, precisely such tension is an indispensable prerequisite of mental health. There is nothing in the world, I venture to say, that would so effectively help one to survive even the worst conditions as the knowledge that there is a meaning in one's life.
> —Viktor Frankl[1]

> Don't aim at success. The more you aim at it and make it a target, the more you are going to miss it. For success, like happiness, cannot be pursued; it must ensue, and it only does so as the unintended side effect of one's personal dedication to a cause

greater than oneself or as the by-product of one's surrender to a person other than oneself. Happiness must happen, and the same holds for success: you have to let it happen by not caring about it. I want you to listen to what your conscience commands you to do and go on to carry it out to the best of your knowledge. Then you will live to see that in the long-run success will follow you precisely because you had forgotten to think about it.

—Viktor Frankl[1]

Reference

1. Frankl V. *Man's Search for Meaning*. Beacon Press; 2006.

Lesson 61
Search for Your Passion and Follow It (Gnaw Your Own Bone)

In choosing an area of medicine to pursue for specialization, it is necessary to see where you find joy. One mentor of mine advised me to look for a domain in which I "enjoyed the plumbing." By this he meant that I should work in an area where I appreciated what was done on a daily basis. If you would like to be a psychiatrist but don't enjoy talking to people, it will not be a good choice. If you would like to be a surgeon but find the operating room boring, terrifying, or both, surgery will not be a good choice. The situation would be different in both cases if you love to talk to people or find the operating room to be continuously exciting and interesting.

American author Henry David Thoreau said, "Pursue, keep up with, circle round and round your life, as a dog does his master's chaise. Do what you love. Know your own bone; gnaw at it, bury it, unearth it, and gnaw it still."[1] Some may be offended with the idea that you should have an interest in your chosen field similar to the interest of a dog for her bone, as suggested by Thoreau. I find his comment very pertinent, perhaps because of my own relationship with a dog.

In the 1990s, I acquired a 6-week-old Chesapeake Bay retriever puppy. This breed is similar in size to a Labrador but has a tremendous innate affinity for water. When the puppy was shown her first water bowl, she climbed into it. In winter, she would do her best to break through the ice to get to the water, and she would have frozen to death if I hadn't pulled her out. This breed has an oily coat and webbed toes. The affection the dog had for water could not possibly be cultural or educational. It could not have been passed down verbally, and it had to be due to her genes and the many generations of selective breeding that produced her affection for water. A genetic influence strongly affecting behavior is produced by many genes and their interactions, not by a single gene.

Undoubtedly many of us have unique preferences which are of genetic origin. These genetically determined affinities are not necessary inherited, as they are the result of a unique combination ig genes which cannot be transmitted from one generation to another. These attributes are not right or wrong. Some people love the water and are happiest when they are on a boat. I like to get on a boat, but not as much as I like to get off a boat. These individual proclivities are a fundamental feature of who we are. It is valuable for each one of us to examine our own lives to see what it may be that provides us the most joy and meaning (Lesson 60).

On the very first day of my surgery clerkship in medical school I showed up at 7 AM and was assigned to a surgical intern who proceeded to lead me in a workday that progressed for more than 20 hours, until 3 AM the next day, with little time for rest or meals. At that time, when our work appeared to be over, we went by elevator to the rooms where we could lie down and sleep for a few hours before the next day's work began. When we reached the floor of the on-call rooms, the elevator doors opened and a stretcher was brought in led by two residents who proceeded to yell "85-year-old ruptured abdominal aneurysm, we're going to the OR." My heart sank as I wondered if I could survive much longer without rest. The surgical intern literally jumped up and down in the elevator saying excitedly, "Oh what a great case, what a great case!" This event was good evidence that a surgical career for me was not advisable.

Your affinity for a specialization either clinical or scientific must be evaluated in regard to aptitude. If you have poor vision, a career in pathology may not be advisable. If you do not have excellent fine motor coordination, a vocation in surgery is not the best choice. If you feel your initial choice may not be best, consider changing your focus. The career of Shinya Yamanaka is an interesting example of changing fields (see below).

Keep in mind that attitudes change. Your initial response to a situation may not be reliable. When I was in college, an uncle of mine worked as a medical examiner in New York City. He took me to see the municipal morgue, which had five autopsy tables, all operating at the same time. I recall being in a state of shock for the entire morning because I had never seen a corpse before. We went out for lunch and when we came back I had adapted and no longer found myself disturbed by the tragic environment. People are extraordinarily adaptive creatures, and it's possible that your initial responses to various situations may not be informative of your genuine nature. The only solution I can think of is to get as much exposure as possible. Pursue opportunities to learn about your options with ferocity (Lesson 4).

> It is quite simple: put passion ahead of training. Feel out in any way you can what you most want to do in science, or technology, or some other science-related profession. Obey that passion as long as it lasts. Feed it with the knowledge the mind needs to grow.
>
> —Edward O. Wilson[2]

> Success is not the key to happiness. Happiness is the key to success. If you love what you are doing, you will be successful.
>
> —Attributed to Albert Schweitzer

Shinya Yamanaka (1962–): A Person to Know

Yamanaka is a Japanese stem cell scientist. He completed his residency in Osaka, Japan, in orthopedics, but he realized that he was not a talented surgeon. He moved to a research position in Kyoto, where he led a group that generated the first induced pluripotent stem (iPS) cells from mouse fibroblasts in 2006. He won the 2012 Nobel Prize in Physiology or Medicine "for the discovery that mature cells can be reprogrammed to become pluripotent." (*Pluripotent* means that an immature or stem cell can give rise to many different cell types.)

References

1. American Reader. 1848. Henry David Thoreau to Harrison Blake, this day in lettres. The American Reader. https://theamericanreader.com/27-march-1848-henry-david-thoreau-to-harrison-blake/ Accessed Nov 3, 2023.
2. Wilson EO. *Letters to a Young Scientist*. Liveright Publishing; 2013.

Lesson 62
Learn to Critically Read the Literature

It is not possible to read everything. Thus, your ability to use your time effectively is important. I suggest receiving the table of contents of the leading journals that are of interest to you. This would certainly include *Nature* and *Science*, and others depending on your background and plans. If you read the titles of all the papers and learn all the words in the titles which you do not know you will enhance your education greatly. Then, of course, you can read the abstracts of interest to you and, if your curiosity is great, read the article. You do not necessarily need to read the entire article. The completeness of your reading will depend on your interest.

If you come upon an article a few years old or much older, you can search for more recent articles that have cited that paper. In this way, you can learn what work followed the original work. Depending on the nature of your interest in the work you may choose to skip reading the methods section. However, it's important to realize that often the methods section is the most important part of the paper.

There are many valuable suggestions on how to manage your reading activities.[1,2] Dr. T. Sun of New York University suggests distinguishing between passive and active reading. *Passive reading* is reading word to word from beginning to end, and *active reading* is reading with questions in mind and searching for answers. The process of active reading will help you remain engaged in the reading process.

To understand the complex figures that are frequently presented in scientific journals it will help to enlarge the figures on your computer so that a graph that occupies perhaps 3 square centimeters on the page is enlarged so that you can clearly see the data. It is easier to focus your attention on a larger area of space.

In an article, "10 simple rules for reading a scientific paper," Carey et al. suggest asking six questions about each paper you read.[3]

> Why was the work done?
> How was it done?
> Why was it done in that way?
> What do the results show?
> What do the results mean?
> What should be done next?

It can be valuable to read books as well as journal articles. Be aware that it takes at least a year or more to publish a book. Therefore, a chapter in a recently published book may be 1 to 2 years out of date, or more.

Consider both what the authors have said in the paper and what they have not said. There may have been things left out because the authors thought they were not important, or perhaps there was not enough space, or the editor did not want them included, or the authors wished to hide something that they want to use for another paper. Perhaps they found something but were not ready to let it be known.

Be critical. Are the results supported by the data? Is the reasoning in the introduction and discussion of the paper reasonable? Has the investigation been influenced by any of the forms of bias discussed earlier? Was the investigation influenced by the sources of support?

Are the findings significant? The P value of <0.05 is entirely arbitrary in determining significance. The P value only informs us about how likely the researchers would it have been to obtain the same results by chance. Remember *statistical significance* is not the same as *clinical significance*: if the number of participants in the study is large enough, a statistically significant finding can very well be meaningless.

Consider this fictional scenario: in a study of a drug intended to enhance memory, 1,000 participants in group A received the active drug, and 1,000 participants in group B received a placebo. The memory test evaluated the number of words remembered after 30 minutes from a list of 20 words. Results show that, in Group A, the mean number of words remembered is 12.42 and in Group B the mean number of words remembered is 12.32. Statistical analysis shows that the recall in Group A is better by one-tenth of a word, with a p value of <0.01. In this fictional scenario, the drug has a statistically significant influence on recall, but the difference is certainly not meaningful or clinically significant.

References

1. Sun TT. Active versus passive reading: How to read scientific papers? *Natl Sci Rev*. 2020 Jun 19;7(9):1422–7. doi:10.1093/nsr/nwaa130. PMID: 34691538; PMCID: PMC8288757.
2. Osler W. A way of life and address to Yale students (1913). ReadaClassic.com; 2010. 9781477642542. Accessed Aug 2024.
3. Carey MA, Steiner KL, Petri WA Jr. Ten simple rules for reading a scientific paper. *PLoS Comput Biol*. 2020 Jul 30;16(7):e1008032. doi:10.1371/journal.pcbi.1008032. PMID: 32730251; PMCID: PMC7392212.

Lesson 63
We Are All Neurologists

We all have a liver, a heart, and kidneys. Our daily life does not inform us well about the function of these organs. The brain is different; our daily life is an expression of neurological activity. There is no aspect of our experience that is not neurological. Our sleep is managed by the brain as well as our alertness, attention, perception, language, judgment, movement, and all other features of our human selves.

A neurologist is a person who is concerned with the function of the nervous system. I propose that all the readers of this book are neurologists because they are also concerned with the function of their brains, as our role in the world is a completely neurological interaction.

There are countless examples of this truth. We learned early in life that if we sit for a long time with our head resting on our hand with our elbow on a table, we will develop pain in the elbow, which shoots down to the hand. This is caused by pressure on the ulnar nerve, which causes its fibers to fire, causing pain in the area of distribution of the sensory fibers of the nerve. If we walk around in the dark at home and smack a toe into an item of furniture, we may notice that the first thing we observe is the feeling of the touch of the toe with the furniture, as well as the sound of the impact. The pain usually follows after a delay of 1/2 to 1 second. Several times I have hit my toe in this manner and immediately concluded that I did not hurt myself because I felt no pain, but was surprised when the pain came a fraction of a second later. This phenomenon is caused by the sound of the impact traveling from my foot to my ear quickly at the speed of sound. The feeling of the toe hitting the object also travels quickly, through touch fibers which involve only two synapses to go from my toe to the brain. The pain fibers, on the other hand, travel more slowly because they are largely unmyelinated (myelin provides insulation to our axons, which allows for faster conduction). Furthermore, the transmission via pain fibers involves more synapses than the sensation of touch. These two examples are given as an illustration of how daily phenomena teach us something about the nervous system.

The same thing can be true concerning observations of how we are affected when we become intoxicated with alcohol or suffer from lack of sleep. Furthermore, everyone who has had success in school has learned how they learn. We learn about the world and about ourselves directly through our observations about our own brain function. Humor is another activity dependent on the brain (see below).

There is another aspect of medicine in which we are all neurologists. All physicians must deal with the patient's capacity for memory, understanding, perception, and learning. If a physician instructs a patient about the use of insulin, she must be aware of the patient's ability to understand the instructions and carry them out because the misuse of insulin may be fatal.

Daily life provides us with the opportunity to learn about how the brain works. The perspective that we are all neurologists can assist in our learning and in our ability to be understanding. We are all specialists in the unique features of our own brains. Realization of these aspects of our selves will enhance our learning and capacity for compassion.

> A sense of humor is just common-sense dancing.
> —Attributed to William James

> When is a little girl not a little girl? When she is a little hoarse.
> —John Hughlings Jackson, British neurologist (from a presidential address he gave to the Medical Society of London on the psychology of joking, 1887).

> Humor activates more brain regions than does information shared without humor.
> —Jason Coronel, American professor of communication[2]

John Hughlings Jackson (1835–1911): A Person to Know

Jackson was a British neurologist who greatly contributed to the scientific advance of neurology. He enhanced the concept of localization of function in the nervous system and provided the first key understanding of focal epilepsy (the Jacksonian march), which he erroneously considered to be a chemical and not an electrical phenomenon. His work established the evolutionary basis of brain function and described how signs and symptoms can result from the release of lower levels from the control of higher levels. Jackson's technique of neurological examination and precise analysis of symptoms and signs helped to establish the discipline of neurology. His work was entirely dependent on his outstanding powers of observation and analysis based on his clinical experience.[1]

References

1. York GK, Steinberg DA. An introduction to the life and work of John Hughlings Jackson with a catalogue raisonné of his writings. *Med Hist Suppl.* 2006;(26):3–157. PMID: 17361913.
2. Coronel JC, et al. Political humor, sharing, and remembering: Insights from neuroimaging. *J Comm.* Feb 2021;71(1):129–161. https://doi.org/10.1093/joc/jqaa041

Lesson 64
Neurology and Cardiology (Etc.) Don't Exist

All of the disciplines of science are artificial. They're valuable but not perfect. It's important to realize that they are concepts and not things; they actually don't exist. Furthermore, there is no region of the brain which is independent of other regions, and there is no part of the body which is independent of other areas. There is a real danger that the power of the disciplines will obscure the reality of the complexity of our existence.

Don't overspecialize. It is necessary that you become a good physician before you become a good super-specialist. Your responsibilities are primarily to the patient and not only to that part of the patient which is your subspecialty.

Human endeavors should not be chopped up into neat cabinets appropriate for long-term storage. Not only are the so-called disciplines of science fictional, but the overlap with nonscientific areas is also vast. Entomologist Edward Wilson has outlined these concepts in his *Letters to Young Scientists*.[1] He says "By pleasure drawn from discovery of new truths, the scientist is part poet, and by pleasure drawn from new ways to express old truths, the poet is part scientist. In this sense science and the creative arts are fundamentally the same." This truth applies as well to physicians as it does to scientists. Enhancing your understanding and appreciation of literature will help you to be a better doctor.

Do not think that because you are a dermatologist, for example, that you do not need to pay attention to medications a patient takes for a bleeding disorder. If you are a psychiatrist, you need to be aware that endocrine disturbances can cause depression as well as psychosis, hallucinations, and delusions. It could be valuable for a psychiatrist seeing a patient with depression to inquire about changes in skin and hair, constipation, fatigue, or altered heart rate, which can be warning signs of endocrine disease. If you are an orthopedist seeing a patient for ankle pain who also complains of ear pain, you should look in the ear and see if there is any pathology evident as well as consider referral to a primary medical doctor or an otolaryngologist.

A valuable word regarding the error of considering the disciplines (or other concepts) to really exist is "reification," the process or result of regarding something abstract as a material or concrete thing. We need to be aware that words are only tools. They represent reality, and they can influence thought in many surprising ways. This is demonstrated in the Buddhist proverb "Do not confuse the moon with the finger pointing at the moon." If you wish to demonstrate the moon to a child you cannot bring it down to show them, you can only point at it. Similarly, words are guides and not actually the thing itself.

A related issue arose in my neurology department. A 45-year-old woman came in with rapidly progressive dementia and evidence on the MRI scan that indicated she may have paraneoplastic limbic encephalitis. This is a form of brain dysfunction caused by antibodies generated by cancer; the antibodies attack the brain, causing cognitive impairment and other abnormalities. The cancer that is responsible for producing the antibodies may be apparent or hidden (occult). This patient had no evidence of cancer, and a CT scan of the chest, abdomen, and pelvis was normal. A whole-body positron emission tomography (PET) scan of glucose metabolism was scheduled. I asked the neurology resident responsible for her care if he had examined her breasts, because breast cancer could be a cause of her condition. He said that it was not necessary because she had had the CT scan of the chest and that he was a neurologist and could not examine breasts. I explained that the false-negative rate of CT scan for breast cancer was greater than zero (a false-negative result occurs when a test indicates that a condition is absent when it is present), that palpation of the breasts takes about 5 minutes and has no side effects and no radiation, and that any doctor should be able to perform it. I also encountered a neurology resident who refused to palpate a patient's testicles because they had been evaluated by a CT scan. A similar situation occurred during my stay in Japan. Imaging does not replace the benefit of the physical examination!

Another example of the dangers of reification occurred in a faculty meeting in my School of Medicine. A proposal was entertained to change the name of the Department of Biochemistry and Molecular Biology to the Department of Biochemistry and Molecular Genetics. I voted against the change because I felt that the word "biology" includes genetics, and retaining the word "biology" is a valuable reminder that all of us are devoted to the study of living things. I was outvoted.

> Do not say, "It is morning," and dismiss it with a name of yesterday. See it for the first time as a new-born child that has no name.
>
> —Rabindranath Tagore[2]

> There are, in truth, no specialties in medicine.
>
> —William Osler[3]

References

1. Wilson EO. *Letters to Young Scientists*. W.W. Norton; 2013.
2. Tagore R. *Stray Birds*. https://poets.org/poem/stray-birds-233-237, accessed Aug. 2024.
3. Osler W. *Acquanimitas*. Ravenia Books; 1937.

Lesson 65
Do Not Respect Boundaries, Be a Trespasser

Yes, there are important boundaries that must be respected. Do not drive under the influence of alcohol or through a red traffic light. Do not perform surgical procedures if you are not trained and experienced in their completion. Otherwise, consider the reality that knowledge does not come in precise buckets, and the brain does not have specific cortical localization for one kind of knowledge that is completely independent from other kinds of knowledge. Consider, where might the border be between chemistry and physics? How about between neurology and psychiatry? All disciplines are arbitrary distinctions which are conceptual and not actual.

This approach to science was well stated by the student of animal behavior Wolfgang Kohler (1887-1967), who said, "It would be interesting to inquire how many times essential advances in science have first been made by the fact that the boundaries of special disciplines were not respected.... **Trespassing is one of the most successful techniques in science**" (emphasis added).[1]

In my career, I have trespassed several times: from neurology to radiology, microbiology, nutrition, genetics, and history. It is a joy to explore new things!

Undoubtedly a great problem in modern medicine is overspecialization. Do you know of the specialist who learned more and more about less and less until she knew absolutely everything about nothing? Many workers in medicine and science reside in silos and know very little about anything other than their own limited topic. If you are able to get out of your silo and look into the silos of others, you may find magnificent opportunities for advancement. Developments in one area may very well be of interest to people in other areas—this a key principle of the history of science.

The fluidity of boundaries can also be applied to psychological factors. The psychiatrist Roy Grinker said, "One can learn more about interrelations between somatic and psychic or between psychic and social systems by making observations at *the boundaries of their intersections*."[2] This supports the need for a multidisciplinary approach looking at somatic factors (relating to the body) as well as psychological and social ones.

Trespassing is a valuable tool for scientific exploration. I recommend it.

> Nature uses only the longest threads to weave her patterns, so each small piece of her fabric reveals the organization of the entire tapestry.
>
> —Richard Feynman[3]

References

1. Kohler W. *Dynamics in Psychology: Vital Applications of Gestalt Psychology.* Liveright; 1940: 115–16.
2. Ghaemi SN. *The Rise and Fall of the Biopsychosocial Model.* Johns Hopkins University Press; 2010.
3. Feynman R. *Messenger lectures.* Cornell University; 1964.

Lesson 66
Be Grateful

All of us in medical and scientific professions have many reasons to be grateful. We have an opportunity to serve others, and we have work that is filled with meaning which is important to other people. The need for our contributions will never be extinguished. We have the magnificent opportunity to live lives filled with meaning. This presents us with an outstanding and long-lasting opportunity to experience gratitude, which is linked strongly to happiness (38). The more that we experience gratitude the happier we will be and the more joy we will experience. Our experience of gratitude, joy, and happiness will make us better physicians who are more able to understand what is happening with our patients. Also, gratitude is a valuable antidote to stress. Stress is a fact of life with which we must all deal (Lesson 72). To be of service to others is a great honor and source of joy. Appreciate it.

The profession of medicine is extraordinarily stable. Only about 5% of American medical students do not graduate. The equivalent rate for engineering students in the United States is 40–50%. In addition, there are a great number of unfilled jobs for doctors, and it is rare to find a physician who cannot find a job. (Recent data suggest that some specialties may face excess supply.) The situation is quite different for engineering, law, music, and many other fields of endeavor where there are relatively few openings compared to the volume of applicants. Workers in the health professions have many reasons to be grateful.

The importance of gratitude is expressed by Bengali Nobel Laureate poet Rabindranath Tagore: "I slept and dreamt that life was joy. I awoke and saw that life was service. I acted and behold, service was joy."

> This is the true joy in life: being used for a purpose recognized by yourself as a mighty one, being a force of nature instead of a feverish, selfish little clod of ailments and grievances, complaining that the world would not devote itself to making you happy. I am of the opinion that my life belongs to the whole community and as long as I live, it is my privilege to do for it what I can, it is a sort of splendid torch which I have got hold of for the moment and I want to make it burn as brightly as possible before handing it on to future generations.
> —Attributed to George Bernard Shaw[1]

I slept and dreamt that life was joy. I awoke and saw that life was service. I acted and behold, service was joy.

—Rabindranath Tagore

Cultivate the habit of being grateful for every good thing that comes to you, and to give thanks continuously. And because all things have contributed to your advancement, you should include all things in your gratitude.
—**Attributed to Ralph Waldo Emerson**

Reference

1. Shaw GB. *Man and Superman*. Dodd, Mead; 1903.

Lesson 67
Look Beyond the Easiest Options and Pursue the Best Resources Possible

Solomon Carter Fuller was an African American neurologist and psychiatrist, born in 1872, in Liberia in West Africa.[1] His paternal grandfather and grandmother were both slaves in Virginia; they emigrated from there to Liberia in 1852. In 1897, he graduated from the Boston University School of Medicine. He was doing postmortem examinations in Boston and was interested in discovering connections between abnormal behavior and the brain. His wish was to obtain training in this area so that he could further his career. He applied for a position with Alois Alzheimer, who was working in the Royal Psychiatric Hospital in Munich, Germany, under the direction of Emil Kraepelin. At that time this was one of the most advanced neuropsychiatry laboratories in the world. He went to Germany for an interview for the job and was accepted by Alzheimer over several German applicants. I greatly admire the courage of Fuller to go to Germany for training. I also admire the open mindedness of Alzheimer to accept him as a colleague.

Frederick Lewy (1885–1950) was a native of Berlin, Germany, and a relative of Paul Ehrlich, recipient of the Nobel Prize in 1908 for contributions to immunology.[2] Lewy studied neuroanatomy with Constantin von Monakow in Zurich and trained in neuropathology with Franz Nissl, Alois Alzheimer, and Walther Spielmeyer in Munich. He studied neurology with Herman Oppenheim in Berlin and psychiatry with Emil Kraepelin in Munich. Remarkably, his mentors included many of the top scientists in Europe in neuropsychiatry. The second leading cause of dementia (after Alzheimer's disease) is named Lewy body disease in his honor.

Note that Thoreau, in the quote below, recommends "advance(ing) confidently in the direction of [your] dreams." This advice can be implemented by seeking the best opportunities available for your education, training, and experience, as illustrated by Fuller and Lewy.

Thoreau recommends building castles in the air and placing their foundations later. I treasure this idea, as many of my teachers would have insisted on building the foundations first. It is best to use your imagination to solve problems and make plans. Don't limit your imagination with limits that may not exist. The work of Alfred Wegener is a good example of this idea. He was criticized for proposing that the continental plates moved because he could not explain the mechanism of this movement (Lesson 80).

I learned this, at least, by my experiment: that if one advances confidently in the direction of his dreams, and endeavors to live the life which he has imagined, he will meet with a success unexpected in common hours. He will put some things behind, will pass an invisible boundary; new, universal, and more liberal laws will begin to establish themselves around and within him; or the old laws be expanded, and interpreted in his favor in a more liberal sense, and he will live with the license of a higher order of beings. In proportion as he simplifies his life, the laws of the universe will appear less complex, and solitude will not be solitude, nor poverty poverty, nor weakness weakness. If you have built castles in the air, your work need not be lost; that is where they should be. Now put foundations under them.
—Henry David Thoreau, *Walden*

A woman's reach should exceed her grasp.
—Robert Browning (adapted)

Solomon Carter Fuller (1872–1953): A Person to Know

Fuller was an African American pathologist who published, with Alzheimer, the first papers on Alzheimer's disease in English. He clarified the pathology of the disease and defined the amyloid plaques and neurofibrillary tangles that are the structural biomarkers of the disease. He had a distinguished career in pathology at Boston University. The Fuller Middle School in Framingham was named after him and his wife, the sculptor Meta Fuller, in 1998.[1] A book about him and his wife, *Where My Caravan Has Rested*, is highly recommended.[1]

References

1. Kaplan M. *Solomon Carter Fuller: Where My Caravan Has Rested*. University Press of America; 2005.
2. Holdorff B. Friedrich Heinrich Lewy (1885–1950) and his work. *J Hist Neurosci*. 2002 Mar;11(1):19–28. doi:10.1076/jhin.11.1.19.9106. PMID: 12012571.

Lesson 68
Focus, but Not Too Much

All kinds of scientific work require focus. You cannot study everything. In the nineteenth century, it was possible to be a "naturalist" and study plants, animals, rocks, and their interactions. Such a generalized approach is difficult today, and you do need to narrow your point of attention so you can make significant contributions. Be careful about being too narrowly focused. We know about the danger of not seeing the forest for the trees. How about not seeing the trees for the leaves? Or not seeing the leaves for the cells, or not seeing the cells for the organelles?

Let's say you become a world expert in technique X. You read everything you can about it, and you ignore other related techniques. You may lose the opportunity for cross-fertilization through your unawareness of what's happening with different methods. And if a new technique replaces the one that is your expertise, you will be left behind.

I had a patient with bismuth poisoning years ago (Lesson 10).[1] At a meeting I met a friend from Newcastle in the United Kingdom who was a specialist in the toxic effects of metals on the brain. I hoped he could help me with this case, but was disappointed that he only knew about aluminum and not any other toxin. I referred a friend in New York with a thyroid problem to a thyroid clinic at a major medical center and was frustrated that she was not offered an appointment because they only dealt with hyperthyroidism and she had hypothyroidism.

Excessive focus will limit your ability to learn from related developments in other fields. Determining where the border is between excessive or inadequate focus is difficult. It is usually best to remember the teaching of Gautama Buddha who advised us of the middle road. As he said, if the strings on a lute are wound too tightly, they will break, and, if they are too loose, they will not sound. He recommended looking for the middle road. Albert Szent-Györgi has a powerful anecdote about what happened to him when he failed to consider the "middle road."

Nobel laureate Albert Szent-Györgi wrote,

> Any level of organization is fascinating and offers new vistas and horizons, but we must not lose our bearings or else we may fall victim to the simple idea that any level of organization can best be understood by pulling it to pieces, by a study of its components—that is, the study of the next lower level. This may make us dive to lower and lower levels in the hope of finding the secret of life there. This made, out of my own life, a wild-goose chase. I started my experimental work with rabbits, but I find rabbits too complex, so I shifted to a lower level and studied bacteria;

I became a bacteriologist. But soon I found bacteria too complex and shifted to molecules and became a biochemist. So I spent my life in the hunt for the secret of life.... The more I knew, the less I understood; and I was afraid to finish my life without knowing everything and understanding nothing. Evidently something very basic was missing. I thought that in order to understand I had to go one level lower, to electrons, and—with graying hair—I began to muddle in quantum mechanics. So I finished up with electrons. But electrons are just electrons and have no life at all. Evidently on the way I lost life; it had run out between my fingers.[2-4]

Clearly Szent-Györgyi was not thinking about the middle road when he decided to "hunt for the secret in life" using electrons as a tool.[3] His essay "Lost in the Twentieth Century" is worth reading [(3)] p. 181.

See also Lesson 61 for a discussion of focus in clinical specialization.

References

1. Friedland RP, Lerner AJ, Hedera P, Brass EP. Encephalopathy associated with bismuth subgallate therapy. *Clin Neuropharmacol*. 1993 Apr;16(2):173–6. doi:10.1097/00002826-199304000-00010. PMID: 8477413.
2. Nobel Prize Organization. Albert Szent-Györgyi: Biographical. Nobel Prize Outreach AB. Oct 17, 2023. https://www.nobelprize.org/prizes/medicine/1937/szent-gyorgyi/biographical./
3. Szent-Györgyi A. Lost in the 20th century. *Ann Rev Biochem*. 1963;32:1–15. https://doi.org/10.1146/annurev.bi.32.070163.000245
4. Szent-Györgyi A. Dionysians and apollonians. *Science*. 1972 Jun 2;176(4038):966. doi:10.1126/science.176.4038.966. PMID: 17778411.

Lesson 69
Be Persistent and Tenacious

It is widely and erroneously believed that the key to academic accomplishment is brilliance. It can be more truthfully stated that the key to accomplishment in any area is hard work. Louis Pasteur is quoted as saying, "**Let me tell you the secret that has led me to my goal: my strength lies solely in my tenacity.**" I find this particularly powerful since he made so many contributions and his work was so unprecedented. Viruses were completely unknown when he developed his vaccines. The nature of the immune response to vaccinations, which provides adaptive immunity to infections, was also unknown. Despite these great handicaps he was able to develop vaccines for anthrax, rabies, and cholera.

It may be that truly brilliant persons are less likely than others to make great contributions because they may not have to work hard to succeed in school. Some people can excel in school with little effort because of prodigious memory and skill in taking exams. But these skills will not serve to advance their accomplishments beyond school. It is hard work which is the true determinant of success.

Your patients and their families will appreciate the thoughtful persistence of your care, and your expression of concern and interest in their welfare needs to be consistent and continuous. Morris Bender, an influential teacher of mine, was well loved by his patients because he would demonstrate his care throughout the course of an illness.

It is worth remembering that your job as a physician is to care for the patient regardless of the effectiveness of the therapy. Hopefully, the patient can be cured and never need see you again. If that is not the case, you are still obliged to care for them. I saw a patient with Alzheimer's disease who had previously seen a prominent neurologist (Dr. X). I asked the patient's wife what Dr. X said about him. She told me that he did not tell her anything about her husband's diagnosis. She called to make another appointment and was told by the nurse that Dr. X said that her husband had Alzheimer's and that he didn't need to come back. This is wrong for several reasons. First, bad news should not be given over the phone, except in unusual circumstances. Second, a physician cannot abandon a patient because the patient has been diagnosed with an illness that cannot be treated effectively. Even in that unfortunate circumstance, the patient and their family need care and concern throughout the disease course.

The situation is similar in scientific endeavors, of course. Research is difficult because you are trying to learn something new. If you wanted to learn something that was already known you could get it from Google, from Chat GTP (a language model-based artificial intelligence system) or countless other sources. Medical research is an internationally diverse effort to learn new things about the body and disease. It is difficult and complex by its very nature. Scientific advances require persistent, concentrated efforts. As expressed by Pasteur, the reward frequently goes to those persons who are the most patient and willing to stay with a problem until it has been solved.

The 2023 Nobel Prize in Physiology or Medicine was awarded to Katalin Kariko and Drew Weissman for discoveries concerning the use of messenger RNA for production of vaccines.[1] Their method uses messenger RNA to elicit production of the spike protein of severe acute respiratory syndrome coronavirus 2 (SARS-CoV-2), which stimulates the body to make antibodies. In the initial years of their research, the Nobel laureates suffered widespread antagonism and paper and grant rejections, and Kariko experienced a demotion and pay cut.[2] Their persistence led to success through the development of an innovative method to avoid harmful effects of the mRNA vaccine. Their method was critical for the successful development of vaccines for the 2020–2022 COVID pandemic.

Louis Pasteur (1822–1895): A Person to Know

Louis Pasteur, French chemist and scientist, was the first to determine how bacteria cause disease and show how attenuated infected tissue could be used to make vaccines. He studied an industrial crisis in the production of silk, caused by silkworm infections, to identify the agent responsible. He improved the production of beer and wine and described the process of fermentation as a biological process for the first time. He was expert in what we call today "technology transfer," when scientific information can be moved rapidly from the laboratory to industry for the benefit of mankind. He trained a generation of great scientists and demonstrated enormous courage and determination. At the age of 45, he had a stroke that left him partially paralyzed on the left, but he successfully pursued his work for many decades. An excellent comprehensive biography of Louis Pasteur was published by P. Dubre.[3]

> You didn't have to be brilliant to be a competent doctor, but you do have to be thorough.
>
> —J. Groopman[4]

References

1. Gristwood A. Getting the message right: An interview with mRNA vaccine pioneer Katalin Karikó. *EMBO Rep*. 2023 Nov 6;24(11):e58261. doi:10.15252/embr.202358261. Epub 2023 Oct 19. PMID: 37855740; PMCID: PMC10626440.
2. Offord C, Cohen J. mRNA discovery that paved way for COVID-19 vaccines wins Nobel Prize in Physiology or Medicine. *Science*. October 2023;382(666):22.
3. Dubre P. *Louis Pasteur*. Johns Hopkins University Press; 2000.
4. Groopman J. *How Doctors Think*. Mariner Books; 2008: 179.

Lesson 70
Do Not Be Intimidated by Accomplished Persons in Medicine and Science

One year after the completion of my research fellowship in 1978, I was working as an assistant professor at the University of California, Davis, and found my research opportunities to be limited. Two grant applications were not funded. I had only a handful of publications. A talk being given at the University of California, Berkeley, on positron emission tomography (PET) scanning stimulated my attention. Professor Thomas Budinger described a new PET instrument that his group had built, which had the best spatial resolution anywhere.[1,*] At the end of his talk, I introduced myself to him saying that I was interested in the applications of his new technology. He said that he was very busy but I could come by the following week. When I arrived the following week, he asked if my slides were ready. Apparently, he expected me to give a talk at his lab meeting. I had no slides because I did not know that I was going to be speaking. I discussed Alzheimer's disease and the problems with available imaging techniques. It turned out that he was looking for applications of his new tomograph. I had scientific questions about Alzheimer's disease but no resources. He had resources but needed scientific questions. Our collaboration was initiated by my approach to him following his presentation and his openness to speak with a neophyte. Together we did some of the first PET studies of Alzheimer's disease.[1]

In Albert Szent-Györgyi's wonderful essay about his life, "Lost in the 20th century,"[2] he reports that, in 1926, his work in Germany was not progressing because his leading collaborator died and was replaced by a psychologist who disliked chemistry. Because of this he had to return to Hungary where his research opportunities were poor. He states that for a "farewell to science" he attended the International Physiological Congress in Stockholm and heard the presidential address delivered by Sir Frederick Hopkins.[†] After the lecture, Szent-Györgyi went to talk to Hopkins who told him "Why don't you come to Cambridge.... I will see to it that you get a Rockefeller scholarship," And that is how Szent-Györgyi obtained a position at Cambridge University. Szent-Györgyi won the 1937 Nobel Prize in Physiology or Medicine for the discovery of hexuronic acid, vitamin C,[3] which he named *ascorbic acid* Lesson 84.

---

   [*] PET scanning is a nuclear medicine procedure in which the uptake and clearance of injected radioactive molecules of interest are measured.
   [†] Sir Frederick Hopkins was chair of biochemistry at Cambridge University and won the Nobel Prize in Physiology or Medicine in 1929 for the discovery of growth-stimulating vitamins.

There are, of course, many other examples of how valuable contacts can be made just by speaking out and asking questions.

If you go to a meeting and hear a distinguished professor give a talk before 2,000 people and you have a question, go up to her at the end, after the session has ended, and congratulate her on the excellent talk and ask your question. The possibilities are (1) she will ignore you as not being important enough to talk to, (2) she will talk to you while she looks over your head for other people who are more important to talk to and not answer your question; or (3) she will answer your question, and you will thank her and possibly she will be impressed with your question and you will end up going to work for her. Of course, these are not the only possible outcomes and they are not all equally likely, but they are all worth consideration. So go ahead and ask!

References

1. Friedland RP, Budinger TF, Ganz E, Yano Y, Mathis CA, Koss B, Ober BA, Huesman RH, Derenzo SE. Regional cerebral metabolic alterations in dementia of the Alzheimer type: Positron emission tomography with [18F]fluorodeoxyglucose. *J Comput Assist Tomogr.* 1983 Aug;7(4):590–8. doi:10.1097/00004728-198308000-00003. PMID: 6602819.
2. Szent-Györgyi A. Lost in the 20th century. *Ann Rev Biochem.* 1963;32:1–15. https://doi.org/10.1146/annurev.bi.32.070163.000245
3. Nobel Prize Organization. Albert Szent-Györgyi: Biographical. Nobel Prize Outreach AB. Oct 17, 2023. https://www.nobelprize.org/prizes/medicine/1937/szent-gyorgyi/biographical/

Lesson 71
Accept the Help of Others

Over 20 years ago, I was engaged in research on Alzheimer's disease in Kenya with collaborators from the United Kingdom and Nairobi. Mount Kenya, which is the second tallest mountain in Africa, is located in the area of the country where we were working. With a colleague, we planned an expedition to climb the beautiful mountain to reach the highest point that could be obtained without using ropes (16,354 ft or 4985 m). As we approached the mountain, we discussed whether or not we would have porters. Porters are widely available and cost about $5 a day at that time. I decided that I certainly wanted to use a porter because I do not commonly climb to such elevations and the trek would take all of 3 days. My colleague said that he would not use a porter because he wanted "to show that he could do it himself." I pointed out that if he really wanted to do it himself he should do it without socks. Also, he should cook his own food, make his own pathway, and not follow the trails made by others.

These considerations led me to conclude that **it is never possible for anyone to do something by themselves.** We all are dependent on the thoughts and actions of others. This idea has also been stated by Carl Sagan, who said, "If you wish to make an apple pie from scratch, you must first invent the universe."[1]

It has become increasingly difficult for science to be done by a single investigator working alone. If you have a hypothesis that requires the use of a certain technique that you do not have available, it may be best for you to develop experience and expertise in the technique. However, this may take a considerable amount of time and expense. Another option is to find a collaborator who is already experienced in the method. It is remarkable how frequently people are happy to collaborate.

Similarly, if you have a difficult case and know of a clinician with great expertise in that condition in another city, consider calling her to discuss your case. You will be surprised at how pleased people are to be acknowledged. Despite their accomplishments physicians and scientists are most often honored to have their work and experience recognized.

The need for collaboration has grown greatly in the past few hundred years of medicine and science. This was not always the case, however. Consider *The Canon of Medicine*, an encyclopedia of medicine contained in five books written by one person, Persian physician-philosopher Avicenna (Ibn Sina), which was completed in 1025. It remained an authoritative work for centuries and was used throughout Europe until

---

[1] My hiking partner did choose to use a porter, and I was happy to give my porter a generous tip, as he carried my backpack as well as his own.

the eighteenth century. It was a more concise work in comparison to the 20 volumes on medicine written by Galen of Pergamon (Turkey) (129–216).

William Osler described the *Canon* as "the most famous medical textbook ever written," which remained "a medical bible for a longer time than any other work."[1] Osler himself authored an important text, *The Principles and Practice of Medicine*, which was first published in 1892. The book was translated into many languages and was the most important medical textbook for more than 40 years. It was widely believed that Osler was the last physician who could cover all of medicine by himself. His textbook was followed by that of Russell Cecil (1881–1965). Cecil invited 130 experts to write chapters concerning their special expertise for his textbook, which was published in 1927. The 27th edition was released in 2023.

In the twentieth century, the scope of knowledge in medicine increased enormously and surpassed the ability of any one person to comprehend the whole. Similarly, in science, the amount of information available is accelerating exponentially. Because of the great growth of knowledge about medicine and science we all need to take advantage of collaboration, which allows for greater opportunities for comprehensive study design and interpretation. Accepting the help of others can be a valuable aid to scientific progress. It is important that care be coordinated among all specialists and subspecialists.

Scientific work is increasingly becoming based more on teams rather than on individual principal investigators. In the past 20 years, the median number of authors of a research paper has increased from three to six, and the percentage of single-authored papers has fallen from 34% in 2002 to 2% in 2021.[2] In medicine, it's wise to seek opportunities to utilize the expertise of others.

Avicenna (Ibn Sina) (980–1037): A Person to Know

Avicenna was a Persian physician and philosopher who had important influences on medicine, philosophy, math, astronomy, and chemistry. It is said that he memorized the entire Koran by the age of 10 and became a physician of the Emir at the age of 17. His works were written in Arabic (the language of science at the time) and Persian and later translated into Latin. His contributions affected medicine and science for several centuries. He is considered the father of early modern medicine, and he was a critical figure in the Islamic Golden Age.[3]

> Many ideas grow better when transplanted into another mind than the one where they sprung up[4]
>
> —Oliver Wendell Holmes, Sr.

References

1. Osler W. *The Evolution of Modern Medicine*. Kessinger Publishing; 2004: 71. ISBN 1-4191-6153-9.
2. Choueiry G. Does the number of authors matter? Data from 101,580 research papers. Quantifying Health. https://quantifyinghealth.com/number-of-authors-of-research-papers/. Accessed May 30, 2023.
3. Arya MP. *The Essential Avicenna*. Xulon Press; 2021.
4. Holmes OW. *The Poet at the Breakfast Table*. Houghton, Mifflin; 1872.

Lesson 72
Pay Attention to Your Own Health and Learn How To Deal with Stress

You cannot take care of others and learn effectively if you're not healthy enough to do the work. Pay attention to sleep habits, diet, and activities to reduce stress. Paying attention to your own health will enhance your capacity for critical thinking. Physical exercise produces new neurons in the brain as well as enhances the production of brain growth factors that enhance synaptic complexity.[1] Diverse forms of physical activity involving aerobic activities, strength building, and stretching are all important.

Diet has strong influences on health. A low saturated fat diet with only small amounts of red meat and large amounts of plants is best. It is wise to limit intake of salt and sugar and avoid artificial colors, flavors, and preservatives (many of these additives are known to be carcinogenic). Intake of dietary fiber and fruit, vegetables, nuts, and grains enhances the production of blood cells that are tolerance-inducing; these are called *Treg cells*, and they diminish the overactivity of the immune system. The impact of diet on the gut bacteria and the brain is reviewed in my book.[2]

Stress is unavoidable. We would not like a life without stress because it would not be very interesting. Of course, there are different levels of stress and different durations of stress (e.g., acute or chronic). We all have different responses to different kinds of stress. Public speaking, for example, is stressful for many people and a joyous experience for others. Our attitude is a critical factor in our response to stress.

Meditation is a valuable activity which helps with our attitude to stress.[3] In meditation, the mind is allowed to focus on one thing, such as the breath, without directed thinking. Thoughts are allowed to come, and they are allowed to go. The mind settles down all on its own without the need for active suppression of thought. A regular practice of meditation has many positive effects on blood pressure, depression, and anxiety in response to stress. Valuable books on meditation techniques have been authored by Vietnamese Buddhist monk Thich Nhat Han and the American Buddhist teacher Jack Kornfield,[4,5] in addition to many others.

It is worthwhile to accept opportunities to experience situations that you may find stressful so that you can learn to adapt. For example, consider agreeing to all opportunities for public speaking, including university, hospital, and community events. This provides you with practice that will help you develop your best communication abilities. Also, if you are looking for a new position, it is helpful to get experience in being interviewed.

Be aware that the amount of stress you experience in a situation may change with time. I am concerned that some students decide not to pursue a career in medicine because they do not like to be around sick persons or blood. They need to understand that most persons adapt to these factors eventually.

Physical exercise is also valuable in dealing with stress. Particularly helpful will be exercising in a natural environment. Sleep is also essential to helping us respond well to stress.

It is prudent to be aware of *empathy fatigue* (also called *compassion fatigue*), which can result from mental and physical exhaustion. Caring for others can be physically and emotionally exhausting. Empathy fatigue is most common with professionals who are concerned with the patient's psychological state. However, it can affect any provider dealing with significant patient suffering.[6] Empathy fatigue occurs in the presence of *burnout* (chronic occupational stress which reduces the ability to work). Prolonged exposure to the suffering of others contributes to trauma in oneself.[7] Both negative and positive emotions are "infectious" (i.e., it is depressing to be around depressed persons). Understanding that you are doing the best you can for them will help. It's also valuable to have breaks and the opportunity for physical and social interactions.

The psychological stresses of the provider can include depression, anxiety, and posttraumatic stress disorder. This may be an increasing problem in healthcare because of the prominent need to see patients quickly. Recognizing the signs of empathy fatigue is important because empathy fatigue can lead to enhanced psychological distress, depression, and interference with patient care.

In my many years of caring for persons with various forms of dementia, I have often felt that I suffered from compassion fatigue. It helps me to know that my service is valuable to my patients and families, even if I cannot provide curative remedies. I believe that one of my most valuable contributions is my listening and availability to my patients and families. Every time I leave the room at the end of a visit, I shake the patient's and caregiver's hands and tell them that they can call me at any time. I give them my cell phone number. Many of the things that happened to persons with dementia are so tragic and unpleasant that the caregiver may not have an opportunity to talk about it to anyone. I provide a valuable service by being there and making sure that the patient and caregiver know that I will be there in the future for them. My ability to deal with compassion fatigue was aided by my knowledge that what I was doing was important to others.

I have occasionally told medical students and residents who see patients with me in clinic that I am sorry there is something that I will not teach them. I will not teach them how to leave the room before the patient knows you're leaving. Or, to put it another way, I don't want them to learn to be a "'roller skate rounder' sailing in and out of the room before the patient has had time to discover what created the draft."[8]

My compassion fatigue is also aided by meditation and regular vigorous physical activity. It is also helped by knowledge that I am committed to research. I hope that my work with my collaborators will be of value in contributing to worldwide efforts to define new molecular mechanisms and ways to deal with neurodegeneration.

The bottom line is, pay attention to your own health. You cannot take care of others if you are not healthy enough to do the work. You need to recognize your limits. Overwork can have dangerous effects on your mental and physical health. In Japan, in 2022, newspapers reported that a 26-year-old physician committed suicide after working 200 hours of overtime in 1 month.[9] Mechanisms for avoiding such exploitation need to be developed globally. Seek professional assistance whenever possible.

> The expectation that we can be immersed in suffering and loss daily and not be touched by it is as unrealistic as expecting to be able to walk through water without getting wet.[10]
>
> —Naomi Remen (1938–), American pediatrician

> The great thing, in all education, is to make our nervous system our ally instead of our enemy.[11]
>
> —William James

References

1. Baloh RW. *Exercise and the Brain: Why Physical Exercise Is Essential to Peak Cognitive Health*. Springer Nature; 2022.
2. Friedland RP. *Unaging: The Four Factors That Impact How You Age*. Cambridge University Press; 2022.
3. Pineda A. Building a meditation routine for a more productive, creative and happier scientific life. *Nature*. 2020 Sep 3. doi:10.1038/d41586-020-02537-5. Epub ahead of print. PMID: 32884144.
4. Hanh Thich Nat. *You Are Here: Discovering the Magic of the Present Moment*. Shambala; 2001.
5. Kornfield J. *No Time Like the Present: Finding Freedom, Love, and Joy Right Where You Are*. Atria; 2017.
6. Stebnicki MA. Empathy fatigue: Healing the mind, body, and spirit of professional counselors. *Am J Psychiatric Rehabil*. 2007;10(4):317–38. https://doi.org/10.1080/15487760701680570
7. Hui L, Garnett A, Oleynikov C, Boamah SA. Compassion fatigue in healthcare providers during the COVID-19 pandemic: A scoping review protocol. *BMJ Open*. 2023 May 31;13(5):e069843. doi:10.1136/bmjopen-2022-069843. PMID: 37258070; PMCID: PMC10255032.
8. Westdahl PR. A letter to Jim: Advice to resident, the importance of being aware. *Am J Surg*. 1979 Jul;138(1):2–7. doi:10.1016/0002-9610(79)90234-4.
9. Yeung J, Ishikawa E. Japanese family says young doctor took his life after working 200 hours overtime in a single month. CNN. Aug 23, 2023. https://www.cnn.com/2023/08/23/asia/japan-doctor1suicide-overwork-karoshi-intl-hnk/index.html.
10. Remen R. *Kitchen Table Wisdom*. Riverhead Books; 2006.
11. James W. *The Principles of Psychology*, Ch. 4; 1890.

Lesson 73
Learn from the History of Medicine and Science

The human mind is not divided into compartments for the various disciplines. We can learn about medicine and science from learning about concepts and discoveries in other fields. Expanding our perspective helps to open our minds to other ways to analyze facts, make decisions, ask questions, evaluate theories, and reach conclusions. This approach is valid even if the learning is in a field different from your own. The mind works in a similar way for all the sciences!

Appreciating how people working in other areas think and reason can be of great value and provide potent insights. I believe that the disciplines are all artificial and that, **there is only one kind of science, and that is the study of everything with all available methods** (Lesson 81). Reading about astrophysics, paleontology, or ichthyology may help us to understand things about scientific questions that we are pursuing. A new technique developed to aid the study of the clouds of a moon of Saturn may turn out to be of value in research on human physiology.

I am not suggesting that human pulmonologists (a subspecialty of internal medicine devoted to the lungs) subscribe to a scientific journal devoted to studies of the planet Saturn. My suggestion is that all varieties of science involve the mind, and the opportunity for cross-fertilization must be welcomed.

A pivotal fact is that human genetics has not enhanced the powers of the brain in the past several hundred years. We certainly have much more knowledge today than doctors and scientists had hundreds of years ago. But evolution has not given us better brains for understanding complex situations. It is valuable to see how our medical and scientific ancestors solved difficult problems even though they had limited knowledge and relatively poor techniques. In 1890, Sir Charles Sherrington, accompanied by Charles Roy, showed that blood flow in the brain depends on metabolic activity. This important contribution was achieved using remarkably primitive methods.[1]

An important feature of the history of medicine and science is that it is fun and incredibly interesting. Barry Marshall, the Nobel laureate and discoverer of the role of *Helicobacter pylori* in peptic ulcer disease, tells the story in his Nobel lecture of how he initially failed when he tried to grow the gastric bacteria in culture.[2] Following these failures there was a crisis in the lab and plates that had been aged for 2 days and that were due to be discarded were left over the weekend by accident. It was discovered that the bacteria were indeed growing and culturable because of the accidental delay in discarding the material.

Deep brain stimulation is a treatment now applied to patients with Parkinson's disease (Lesson 93). The idea that physically altering the brain could improve the disease resulted from an unusual stroke in a patient with Parkinson's disease that improved his motor impairment. Initially, brain lesions were induced in patients with Parkinson's disease, but more recently precise areas of brain malfunction can be induced repetitively and temporarily with deep brain stimulation, thus improving motor impairment.

Alexander Fleming often gets credit for the discovery of penicillin (Lesson 82). Even though he was not the first to use microbial products for the treatment of infections, he did appreciate the importance of penicillin. Purification of the antibiotic was not done by Fleming but by scientists at Oxford University, who succeeded in making penicillin into a life-saving drug. This teaches us that it is not the responsibility of each investigator to accomplish all the goals of a project. Through collaboration it may be a possible to achieve aims that appeared to be unattainable.

Emil Kraepelin was a leading figure in early twentieth-century psychiatry. He is best known for his revision of psychiatric diagnosis, design of psychiatric hospitals, studies on drug effects on behavior, views of the nosology of psychiatric disease, and his *Textbook: Foundations of Psychiatry and Neuroscience* (1883) (nosology is the study of disease classification). In 1910, Kraepelin chose his junior faculty member Alois Alzheimer to receive the eponym of presenile dementia in his influential text.[3,*]

Kraepelin's establishment of the disease as a form of dementia occurring before the age of 65 years (presenile) was a grievous error because it led to the neglect of the more common onset of dementia, which occurs after the age of 65. This story illustrates the powerful influence of social factors and the great influence that words have on medical practice.

There are an infinite number of such stories about the remarkable history of discovery.

Emil Kraepelin (1856–1926): A Person to Know

Kraepelin was a German neuropsychiatrist considered to be the founder of modern scientific psychology. He emphasized the biological features of behavioral disorders, in contrast to Sigmund Freud, who emphasized psychodynamic factors. His textbook was used worldwide for several decades. Alois Alzheimer worked in his institute in Munich, and Kraepelin chose to name presenile dementia after Alzheimer in his textbook in 1910 (*presenile* means having an onset before the age of 65, and *dementia* is a complex of symptoms and signs comprised of difficulty with memory and cognition

---

[*] I have proposed that he gave the honor to his own colleague to prevent it going to the Czechs Arnold Pick or Oskar Fischer, who were both Jewish and had both published papers on the pathology of the disease before Alois Alzheimer. Kraepelin's antisemitism was well known because he documented it firmly in a paper called "self-assessment" in 1920.[4]

interfering with social and occupational functioning). Kraepelin advocated for the humane treatment of patients in psychiatric hospitals. Toward the end of his life, he was a proponent of racial hygiene, eugenics, and antisemitism.

A good place to start reading about the history of medicine and science is *Advice for a Young Investigator* by Santiago Ramon y Cajal.[5]

The past is never dead. It's not even past.

—William Faulkner, American novelist[6]

References

1. Friedland RP, Iadecola C. Roy and Sherrington (1890): A centennial reexamination of "On the regulation of the blood-supply of the brain." *Neurology*. 1991 Jan;41(1):10–4. doi:10.1212/wnl.41.1.10. PMID: 1985272.
2. Nobel Prize Organization. Barry Marshall Nobel lecture. 2005. https://www.nobelprize.org/prizes/medicine/2005/marshall/lecture/.
3. Friedland RP. *Unaging: The Four Factors That Impact How You Age*, Cambridge University Press; 2022.
4. Engstrom EJ, Burgmair W, Weber MM. Emil Kraepelin's "self-assessment": Clinical autography in historical context. *Hist Psychiatry*. 2002 Mar;13(49 Pt 1):89–119. doi:10.1177/0957154X0201304905. PMID: 12096750.
5. Ramon y Cajal S. *Cerebrum*. 2016 Sep-Oct:11–16.
6. Faulkner W. *Requiem for a Nun*. Knopf Doubleday reprint edition; Jan 3 2012.

Lesson 74
Recognize Your Intellectual Ancestors

I have thought of putting up a sign at the entrance of a medical school asking everyone entering to remove their shoes. Why? The truth is that all of us practicing medicine and doing science are benefiting from the past several hundred years of scholarship and research. It was Isaac Newton who devised a famous metaphor in a 1675 letter to express this: "If I have seen further [than others], it is by standing on the shoulders of giants." I'm sure that my readers would agree that it would be rude for us to show disrespect to our intellectual ancestors by wearing shoes as we stand on their shoulders.

In all seriousness, our current understanding of the world comes from contributions which have come before. The works of Isaac Newton are well-known, and his influence is well-recognized today. The recipient of his letter was Robert Hooke, who designed one of the first compound microscopes and may have been the first to see microorganisms in 1665. He also coined the term "cell." Clearly the contributions to science made by Newton and Hooke are profound. How about the more recent past?

One fun way of addressing the issue of our dependence on our intellectual ancestors is to consider the *Neurotree figure* (The Neuroscience Academic Family Tree) https://neurotree.org/neurotree/tree.php?pid=609; accessed August 2024. The Neurotree figure shows the history of academic mentoring for each individual. My figure shows that I was a student of Morris B. Bender at the Mount Sinai School of Medicine, who was the student of John Fulton at Yale. And Fulton was a student of C. S. Sherrington at Oxford and Harvey Cushing at Yale. And Sherrington studied with both Rudolf Virchow of Berlin and Robert Koch from Berlin and William Halstead of Johns Hopkins. I have offered this website to my students for many years, and I find that most have little interest in it. I find it meaningful to think that something I teach may have been taught to me by Bender, and he may have learned it from Fulton, who learned from Virchow.

Consideration of our intellectual ancestors also reminds us that they were every bit as human as we are. It is a natural tendency to assume that anyone who could come up with such profound discoveries must be made from unique materials or blessed with pixie dust. However, studies of the lives of these individuals show us that they were all 100% human with human talents, human errors, and all too human misconceptions and deficiencies. A critical conclusion is that it is wrong to think, for example, "Who am I to do cancer research, I am not nearly as smart as Harold Varmus?" (winner of the 1989 Nobel Prize in Physiology or Medicine for discovering cancer-causing viruses). Believe in yourself. You will not know what you can accomplish until you try.

William Halsted (1852-1922): A Person to Know

Halsted was an American surgeon who advanced the use of aseptic techniques, as originally developed by Joseph Lister (Lesson 34). He went to medical school at Columbia University, and, upon graduation, he went to Europe to work with prominent physicians including some of the leading ones in the world at the time. He originated the radical mastectomy for breast cancer and performed early blood transfusions. In the 1880s, he was exposed to cocaine as part of his work and became addicted to both cocaine and morphine. He was a founding professor at the Johns Hopkins Hospital and was an outstanding teacher with several celebrated students, including neurosurgeons Harvey Cushing and Walter Dandy.

Lesson 75
You Are an Educator—That's One of Your Most Important Responsibilities

Nearly all medical and scientific professions require participants to be educators. If you are a fourth-year medical student, you will be called upon to teach students from the earlier years. If you are a resident, you will be responsible for teaching other residents and students. And, critically, throughout your career you will be teaching patients and families. You will be teaching them about their conditions and what they need to do to maintain their health and fitness.

Speaking to patients requires you to realize that information alone is not satisfactory. Everyone knows by now that cigarette smoking causes cancer, heart attacks, strokes, and countless other infirmities. Rather than tell people that they must stop smoking because it has bad effects on their health, you must explain to them what they can do to stop and tell them why and how in a manner that relates best to them individually. Put your advice into the context of their lives (Lesson 3).

Similarly, the most effective teaching you will provide must consider the nature of the audience and instill interest, which will sustain learning beyond the brief time that you may have together. It is worthwhile to take classes and workshops and use opportunities for training in education. Do not assume that you know how to be a good educator because you are intelligent—the two things often do not go together. You must pay attention to your abilities as a teacher, no matter what career you pursue.

A key element in teaching is the transmission of your passion. Whatever you are teaching, you need to communicate your interest in the subject and why it is important. What can the students get from you that they can't get in a textbook? Furthermore, to be an effective teacher of patients and families, you must transmit your concern and interest in their welfare.

Teaching is an important part of your work for many reasons. Much of the costs of medical education and research are supported by the government. We all have an obligation to educate the public in consideration of this support. Also, teaching helps you understand the concepts of your work. There is no better way to advance in your understanding of the matter at hand than to teach. I cannot neglect to mention that teaching is fun and that I'm grateful for the opportunity to learn from my audience.

A remarkable example of learning from an audience occurred when my daughter was in second grade and I volunteered to talk to her class about the brain. I spoke briefly about the brain and then asked the children if they could tell me what the brain does. I was interested in teaching them that the brain does everything. They came up with several reasonable answers, and, when one little girl raised her hand, I asked her what was it that she thought the brain did. She frowned and said "Oh, I forgot" (she forgot what she was going to say). I said "You're right, very good! Forgetting is a function of the brain." I had not previously considered that forgetting is important for memory. If I remembered everywhere I had ever parked my car, it would be difficult to remember where I parked it today. The observation that forgetting is a normal function of the brain helps me explain age-related change in memory to my patients.

Publishing is also a critical component of your teaching. In the clinic, you may be advising a person about his condition. This audience of one person is the fundamental structure of medicine. If you give a talk, you may have an audience of 10, 100, or more depending on the situation. When you write a paper that is subsequently published, you have no idea how many thousands of readers will receive benefit from your contribution. Although your paper may not be devoted to the concept of teaching, it has an educational component nonetheless. Not only will the number of persons exposed to your teaching be greater than with a lecture but you also don't know how long the influence of your paper will last.

Furthermore, writing helps you understand your subject. The need to put concepts into words is the most valuable method for enhancing your understanding. Author William Zinsser says, "Writing is a tool that enables people in every discipline to wrestle with facts and ideas, ... It compels us by the repeated effort of language to go after those thoughts and to organize them and present them clearly. It forces us to keep asking, 'Am I saying what I want to say?' "[1]

Dr. Simmons Lessell was a founder of the field of neuro-ophthalmology and an outstanding educator that I had the good fortune to meet in Boston. Asked in a 2007 interview what made his teaching special, he answered: "I'm honest." "I acknowledge my shortcomings," he told the *Journal of Neuro-Ophthalmology*. "I've also tried to be generous. If you have more pieces of the puzzle than the person you are teaching, the next criterion is generosity. What you are trying to do is to give to someone else everything that you have acquired and the means of gaining more. You hope that each one will do even better than you do. The teacher who holds back or is abusive or gruff—I do not see a place for that."[1]

References

1. Zinssser W. *Writing to Learn*, p 41. Harper Collins; 1993.
2. Lessell S. Simmons Lessell, the goal of neuro-ophthalmology. *J Neuroophthalmol.* 2007 Mar;27(1):61–73. doi:10.1097/WNO.0b013e3180321593. PMID: 17414878.

Lesson 76
Learn To Be a Salesperson

Regardless of what specialty you pursue, you need to be able to convince others of the value of your ideas. Your ability to sell yourself and your concepts is important in teaching students, patients, caregivers, and colleagues. This concept applies as well to scientific papers, presentations, and conferences.

It is critical to understand how people learn and how behavior can be changed. It is best to personalize your guidance whenever possible when instructing patients. For interactions between doctor and patient, information is not enough. You cannot tell them that they are too heavy without helping them make a plan to manage their obesity. Information is also not enough for scientific communications. If you are giving a scientific talk, you cannot expect the audience to pay attention to 40 Western blots shown without interruption (a Western blot is a lab technique for detecting specific proteins). It is necessary to consider the attention span of the audience and the fact that they are unlikely to be as interested in the results as you are.

Public speaking is an important part of medicine and science. Regardless of the nature of your career, you need to be able to speak in public to both physicians and laypersons. There are several resources available to help you learn this important skill. You can inquire at your institution about classes that might be available. Educational sessions on public speaking may also be available in your community. Use every opportunity available to give talks so that you can practice your skills.[1,2]

Get to know your audience so you can address your talk appropriately. One valuable summary of the task of public speaking is that your talk should have three parts: first you tell them what you are going to tell them, then you tell them, and then you tell them what you told them. This over-simplification contains an element of truth. Be sure to look at your audience as you speak, and address your comments to them directly. Do not face the screen, and do not overuse your pointer. It is rude to take up all the time available, as you must leave time for questions. Use the questioning as an opportunity to restate the main issues of your presentation.

It is natural to have anxiety when learning public speaking. Remember that most of the time you will know more about your subject than anyone else in the audience. Many years ago, I was giving one of my first talks to a group of physicians and scientists interested in cerebral blood flow. The developer of the technique I was speaking about was sitting directly in front of me. He looked at me every few minutes during the talk with an expression of concern. As my talk progressed, he was furiously writing notes on a yellow pad, and then he looked up at me with an unhappy expression. I was terrified of what he would say but when I concluded my talk he did not ask any questions. I told him later that I thought he was going to ask me a question because he had been writing so intently during my speech. He said nonchalantly that he has been writing a letter to his brother.

In 1981, I was giving a talk at the Society for Nuclear Medicine's annual meeting on measurement of glucose metabolism in the brain in Alzheimer's disease using positron emission tomography. I was worried that I would be asked about the complex mathematics involved in determining the cerebral metabolic rate for glucose from the imaging data. There were various forms of an equation involved in this calculation which I could not comprehend. At the end of my talk, I was upset to see a distinguished physicist get up to ask me a question. I thought he would ask about my understanding of this important equation. I was shocked when he asked me "What is Alzheimer's disease?"

The best way to deal with the stress of public speaking is through practice. It is a joy to share your knowledge with others.[3]

References

1. Kearns F. *Getting to the Heart of Science Communication: A Guide to Effective Engagement*. Island Press; 2021.
2. Rubenson D. Good presentation skills benefit careers—and science. Career Guide. *Nature*. 2021 Jun;594(7864):S51–S52. doi:10.1038/d41586-021-01281-8.
3. Carnegie D. *Public Speaking for Success: The Complete Program, Revised and Updated*. Penguin; 2006.

Lesson 77
Learn How To Learn from Bad Example

It is best to learn from good example, of course, but this is not always possible. You must master both methods: learning from good as well as bad example. When you attend a conference presentation or a lecture, there are always at least two things you can learn. You can learn about the content of the presentation, and you can also learn about how to give a presentation or how not to give a presentation. I recently attended a scientific lecture with excellent content which was impaired by the speaker, who faced the screen throughout. He had a computer in front of him and could have seen his slides while he faced the audience, but he chose to face the screen, and we could not see his face.

We all wish our teachers were kind, generous, thoughtful, brilliant, caring, and insightful. When they lack these outstanding features, we can still learn from them. Many of the teachers I had in New York City during my medical school and residency taught by using humiliation and embarrassment. Somehow, they decided that students needed to be reminded of how little they knew so they would work harder. If you saw a patient on rounds and suggested the presence of a certain disease, the instructor was likely to respond "Oh, is that right, you think it might be X. Well, tell me how many cases of that have you seen, *professor*?" They rarely complimented the students, and, if a student could answer a question, they would be irritated and ask a harder question. The faculty would keep asking more difficult questions until they had exposed the student's ignorance. I hope that I learned from these experiences the need to be supportive, encouraging, and complimentary when appropriate. Also, I realize that it is necessary for me to be aware of the fact that I wasn't trained in how to teach in a supportive and encouraging manner. Awareness of this deficit in my experience has helped me to be a better educator.

> Example is not the main thing that influences others. It is the only thing.
> —Attributed to Albert Schweitzer

Lesson 78
Remember Pierre Curie, Carl Wernicke, and Others

Pierre Curie (1859–1906) died at the age of 46, crossing a street in Paris when he was run over by a carriage. He was the husband of Marie Curie (nee Sklodowska) and was a recipient of the 1903 Nobel Prize in physics with his wife.

Carl Wernicke (1848–1905) died at the age of 58 years while bike riding in the Thuringian forest of southern Germany. He was a German neuropsychiatrist who produced groundbreaking studies of aphasia and brain disease.

Paul Schilder (1886–1940), psychoanalyst and neuroscientist, died at 54 years of age after being struck by a truck on First Avenue in New York City. He is known as a founder of group psychiatry and has several conditions named after him.

Patricia S. Goldman-Rakic (1937–2003) neuroscientist, died crossing a residential street near her home in Connecticut, at 66 years of age. She made many important advances in understanding the workings of the frontal lobe in humans.

The mental life of physicians and scientists is often active and constantly engaged in thought. You may be going from one hospital building to another thinking about your patients and their response to your care and thus neglect to notice what is happening as you cross the street. Perhaps you are working in your mind to plan your next experiment while you take a shortcut through the parking lot at night. It is an occupational hazard of persons involved in cognitively demanding tasks to be the victims of accidents. In the writing of this book, I have noted that I can be absorbed in the process of writing for hours without awareness of what's going on. While I am driving my car, I may think of something I need to add to the book. Hopefully, I must remember to be always attentive to the road. Regardless of the importance of your thoughts, you need to pay attention to what you're doing!

There is another important reason to remember Carl Wernicke. The brain disease named after him (Wernicke's encephalopathy) is caused by a deficiency of thiamine (vitamin B_1).[1] It may be seen in alcoholics, persons who have had GI surgeries, or other persons who are seriously malnourished. The condition can cause memory loss, dementia, hallucinations, delusions, visual problems, ataxia, and delirium. It is critical that patients suspected of having this problem receive parenteral thiamine administration. (*Parenteral* means "outside of the intestines," such as through the intravenous or intramuscular route.) If the condition is not adequately and urgently treated, permanent severe memory loss or death may result. Studies show that more than 50% of people with Wernicke's encephalopathy are not diagnosed before death.[2]

If thiamine was a drug that could help a drug company make money, we would all be seeing ads on TV about the importance of recognizing thiamine deficiency. However, no one can make a profit from the vitamin, and therefore public awareness of its importance is poor.

I hope that knowing that this great scientist died in a bicycle accident will make us all more attentive to hazardous situations. I am also hopeful that being reminded of his life will help us to remember the importance of thiamine deficiency.

Carl Wernicke (1848–1905): A Person to Know

Wernicke was a German neuropsychiatrist and neuropathologist. He studied the influence of brain lesions on speech and understanding of language and described sensory aphasia, now known as *Wernicke's aphasia*. This was in contrast to the motor aphasia described by Paul Broca in Paris. He also described the effects of thiamine deficiency on the brain, referred to as *Wernicke's encephalopathy*, and he was one of the first to use photography to study brain pathology. His network view of neuronal function was prescient.[3]

References

1. Sachdeva A, Chandra M, Choudhary M, Dayal P, Anand KS. Alcohol-related dementia and neurocognitive impairment: A review study. *Int J High Risk Behav Addict*. 2016 Feb 7;5(3):e27976. doi:10.5812/ijhrba.27976. PMID: 27818965; PMCID: PMC5086415.
2. Wolfe M, Menon A, Oto M, Fullerton NE, Leach JP. Alcohol and the central nervous system. *Pract Neurol*. 2023 Aug;23(4):273–85. doi:10.1136/pn-2023-003817. Epub 2023 Jun 16. PMID: 37328277.
3. Pillmann F. Carl Wernicke (1848–1905). *J Neurol*. 2003 Nov;250(11):1390–1. doi:10.1007/s00415-003-0250-x. PMID: 14648163.

SECTION VI
DISCOVERY

Lesson 79
What Is Science?

According to the *Oxford English Dictionary*, "Science is the state or fact of knowing; knowledge or cognizance of something." The *Cambridge Dictionary* defines science as "[knowledge from] the careful study of the structure and behavior of the physical world, especially by watching, measuring and doing experiments and the development of theories to describe the results of these activities." You see in these definitions the concepts of "fact of knowing" and "careful study," which suggest a rational process.

Is this correct? Is science a rational process? (*Rational* means something which is based on reason and logic.) Science is a tool we use to understand the world and is subject to all the shortcomings of the human mind. Archimedes (287–212 BC) discovered buoyancy when he took a bath and noticed something, then he ran naked through the streets exclaiming "Eureka!" This exemplifies the importance of intuition, a decidedly nonrational process (Lessons 42 and 45).

If science was rational, it should progress from one stage to another in a single series of steps, in a linear fashion. Discovery A leads to B, to C, and so on, and we therefore end up with an understanding of atoms, or DNA, or polymerase chain reactions, or the sequence of human genome. And certainly, there is plenty of apparent evidence for this phenomenon of linear advancement.

But science is not linear and is not rational. For example, evolution is not linear. It does not progress at a constant rate. The discovery of asepsis (the removal of microbes) by British surgeon Joseph Lister (1827–1912) was not the result of a careful series of experiments over years but rather the product of Lister's imagination.[1] About 66 million years ago, an enormous asteroid struck the Yucatan Peninsula, created a 150-kilometer crater, and contributed to the rapid death of many of Earth's life forms, especially dinosaurs. This was decidedly not part of a linear process.

Looking at the past, it appears that science has progressed in a rational and linear manner. This perspective is misleading.

The British writer Arthur Koestler[2] expressed science's nonlinear nature in his *The Act of Creation*, "[Science] advances in a jerky, unpredictable "unscientific" way … if we could take a kind of grandstand view of the history of scientific thought we would be at once struck by its discontinuity, its abrupt changes of tempo and rhythm."

The American philosopher of science Thomas Kuhn (1922–1994) reviewed scientific discoveries and concluded that knowledge does not progress in a rational and linear process, with small discoveries gathering evidence for new theories. He proposed rather that they move suddenly, with rapid developments of new concepts. In his important book *The Structure of Scientific Revolutions* (1962), he developed the term "paradigm shift,"[3] which is a fundamental change "when the usual and accepted way of doing or thinking about something changes completely" (*Cambridge Dictionary*).

Kuhn's colleague at the University of California, Berkeley, Paul Feyerabend (1924–1994) supplemented Kuhn's position that science does not progress through rational or linear processes. In his *Against Method* (1975), he said **"There is only *one* principle that can be defended under *all* circumstances and in *all* stages of human development. It is the principle: anything goes."**[4] He meant that there are no fixed rules, and there is no magical "scientific method." Our imagination in science should not be limited by preconceived ideas. **What is important in science is problem-solving, not conforming to established modes of thought.** Diversity of approaches is critical.

Although both Kuhn and Feyerabend developed their concepts from the study of the history of physics, their thoughts are important for all branches of science. The critical feature of the scientific enterprise is that it is a product of the mind, regardless of what the subject is. Concepts in planetary geology can be of interest to persons studying infant nutrition, for example. The great commonality of all scientific work is that it all depends upon the mind.

There are countless examples in science of the validity of the "anything goes" concept. Let's consider three brief stories for illustration.

The discovery that high doses of levodopa are effective for the treatment of Parkinson's disease was not anticipated. It had been determined in 1960 that, in the basal ganglia, in the disease there was a deficiency of dopamine, and the idea of replacing it with levodopa was considered. Initial trials were negative until Greek neurologist George Cotzias showed that significantly higher doses were effective (1969). It was not known before he tried it that high doses would be affective. He said "the proper dose of dopa is enough to stop the disease."[5]

The transmissibility of kuru and Creutzfeldt-Jakob disease was reported by Daniel Carleton Gadjusek (1923–2008) and colleagues in the 1960s (Lesson 92). It was originally thought that the disease could not be infectious or transmissible because the brain pathology did not show any evidence of infiltration of immune cells. All other transmissible brain diseases at that time, such as bacterial or viral meningoencephalitis, had an excess of immune cells in the brain. It turns out that kuru and Creutzfeldt-Jakob disease are infectious and transmissible but are lacking in the characteristic pathology expected of infectious diseases.[6,7]

In the late eighteenth century, beri-beri was common in Asia where rice is prominent in the diet. The disease causes neuropathy (damage to peripheral nerves), with weakness and numbness in the legs, muscle atrophy, cardiac failure, cognitive problems, and high mortality. A toxic factor in the rice was suspected but could not be identified. Although it was believed that the disease was caused by bacteria, it was not transmissible from humans to animals or from animal to animal. A Japanese Navy doctor, Takaki Kanehiro (1849–1920), eliminated white rice from the diet of the sailors, added nutrient-rich foods, and found that beri-beri was eradicated. Because of the bias that the disease was infectious the discovery was forgotten. Dutch physician

Christiaan Eijkman suggested that the transmission of the disease had a long incubation period, so in his experiments chickens were used because they were relatively inexpensive. The animals were noted to develop a polyneuropathy, with unsteady gait and falling, followed by axonal degeneration of the nerves and death. The disease in the chickens was found to be unrelated to exposure to affected chickens. The lab was in a military hospital, and the technician in charge, on his own initiative, changed the diet from polished (white) rice to unpolished (brown) rice to save money. This change cured the disease in the chickens. Eijkman also noted that beri-beri was more common in people who ate white rice, and he found that the prevalence of the disease in prisons where polished (white) rice was used was 300 times greater than in those where rough (brown) rice was eaten. The anti–beri-beri factor, thiamine (vitamin B_1), was not synthesized until 1936.

Appreciation of the reality that science does not develop by precise rational steps and that "anything goes" is critical for progress in both medicine and science. This can be seen in consideration of great discoveries which involve a "paradigm shift." If Newton's work on gravity or Semmelweis' studies of childbed fever (Lesson 34) could have been the result of small steps they would have occurred centuries earlier. **It is only in retrospect that great discoveries appear to be the result of logical thought.**

The point of view I am suggesting—openness to new ideas—is not easy, but it is both necessary and exciting.

Christiaan Eijkman (1858–1930): A Person to Know

Eijkman was a Dutch military physician who contracted malaria at a young age and developed an interest in tropical medicine. He trained with Robert Koch in Berlin, which may have influenced him to suspect that beri-beri was likely to have an infectious origin. He was thankfully open to learn from planned and unplanned experiments in studies of the disease in humans and animals. Dissemination of his work was limited by his publication in the Dutch language. He also developed an important technique for detecting stool contamination in water supplies. Eijkman won the 1929 Nobel Prize in Physiology or Medicine "for his discovery of the anti-neuritic vitamin."[8]

> I am never happy with the theory until it leads me into a flat contradiction with a fact. Then I know I had a theory.
> —Attributed to Harold Urey (1893–1981), American physical chemist, Nobel laureate, and discoverer of deuterium

> Basic research is what I am doing when I don't know what I'm doing.
> —Attributed to Wernher von Braun (1912–1977), German aerospace engineer

References

1. Fitzharris L. *The Butchering Art: Joseph Lister's Quest to Transform the Grisly World of Victorian Medicine.* Farrar, Straus and Giroux; 2017.
2. Koestler A. *The Act of Creation.* Macmillan; 1964: 226.
3. Kuhn T. *The Structure of Scientific Revolutions.* University of Chicago Press; 1996.
4. Feyerabend P. *Against Method.* Verso; 2020.
5. Cotzias GC, Van Woert MH, Schiffer LM. Aromatic amino acids and modification of parkinsonism. *N Engl J Med.* 1967 Feb 16;276(7):374–9. doi:10.1056/NEJM196702162760703. PMID: 5334614
6. Asher DM, Gregori L. Human transmissible spongiform encephalopathies: Historic view. *Handb Clin Neurol.* 2018;153:1–17. doi:10.1016/B978-0-444-63945-5.00001-5. PMID: 29887130.
7. Gajdusek DC, Gibbs CJ, Alpers M. Experimental transmission of a Kuru-like syndrome to chimpanzees. *Nature.* 1966 Feb 19;209(5025):794–6. doi:10.1038/209794a0. PMID: 5922150.
8. Pietrzak K. Christiaan Eijkman (1856–1930). *J Neurol.* 2019 Nov;266(11):2893–5. doi:10.1007/s00415-018-9162-7. Epub 2018 Dec 26. PMID: 30588543; PMCID: PMC6803585.

Lesson 80
No Single Theory Ever Agrees with All the Facts

> No single theory ever agrees with all the facts in its domain.
> —Paul Feyerabend

The Hungarian American mathematician John von Neumann (1903–1957) said "Truth … is much too complicated to allow anything but approximations." This demonstrates that ideas do not need to be perfect to be valuable. A theory does not need to fit all the data available for its analysis, as stated by Paul Feyerabend in the title of this lesson.[1]

If I had told my genetics teacher in college in the 1960s that I wanted to work on the transfer of human genes to mice, she would have considered me a dunce since the belief was that such transfer was certainly not possible. The idea that human genes could be expressed in animals did not fit with the genetics concepts of the time.

If you have an idea about a clinical or scientific problem and there is evidence that your idea is wrong, there are two chief possibilities: (1) your idea is wrong or (2) your idea is correct and the evidence that your idea is wrong is wrong. Remember the story of *Helicobacter pylori* as a cause of peptic ulcers, which was initially rejected because of the erroneous belief that bacteria could not live in the stomach (Lesson 48). **Remember that all bad ideas have reasons to believe them, causing good ideas to be resisted.**

Feyerabend also said, "Not only are facts and theories in constant disharmony, they are never as neatly separated as everyone makes them out to be."[1] Our minds prefers order, and we often naturally choose simplicity whenever possible. This powerful tendency to reduce complexities into easier-to-understand concepts can be hazardous. We have been warned about this by Albert Einstein, who is often quoted as having said "Everything should be made as simple as possible, but no simpler." What he actually said in 1933 was "It can scarcely be denied that the supreme goal of all theory is to make the irreducible basic elements as simple and as few as possible without having to surrender the adequate representation of a single datum of experience."[2] He is warning us to be careful when we seek simplicity.

Sydney Brenner had a valuable way to conceptualize the fact that new theories do not need to be perfect (Lesson 60). He proposed a "don't worry hypothesis" so that you can go on and evaluate something and "don't have to worry about it at that very moment."³ His example was the original problem with the DNA structure proposed by Watson and Crick: How could the chains be unwound because they were not parallel, but intertwined? This was not originally clear. Brenner postulated enzymes to unwind the strands, which were later documented as DNA helicases.

Consider the sad story of German climatologist Alfred Wegener (1880–1930) who developed the concept of continental displacement, which describes the movement of the outermost layer of the earth (now known as *continental drift* due to plate tectonics). His work was presented in a 1915 publication *The Origin of Continents and Oceans*. He pointed out that continents fit well together, like a couple spooning in bed, if the idea of their movement is considered.⁴ The similarities of plants and animals in locations at the sites where the continents would have been originally joined was also noted. His ideas were criticized as "delirious ravings" because there was no mechanism which would allow for the continents to move, and the idea that the continents were stable in their present positions was well-established. The theory was not accepted until geological discoveries of the 1950s. Wegener died of exposure on an expedition to the center of the Greenland ice sheet in 1930.

The folly of rejecting Wegener's hypothesis shows how it can be hazardous to expect every new idea to explain all of its background and implications. In 1915, geological knowledge could not explain how the continents could move. I can't resist quoting Galileo: "And yet it moves."*

The idea that theories do not need to explain all related phenomena is central to decision-making in science and medicine. Appreciation of the reality that science does not develop by precise rational steps and that "anything goes" is critical for progress in scientific endeavors, including the practice of medicine. Pediatric neurologist David Clark taught me that it was permissible to "throw out" one feature of every case. He did not mean to ignore it, but rather to understand that humans are complex, and it is not necessary for everything to fit perfectly when considering a diagnostic category. If you are considering a diagnosis and one of your findings does not support that diagnosis, that does not mean that the diagnosis cannot be correct. Similarly, imagine that you propose a new idea at a lab meeting and a colleague points out evidence indicating that the idea is wrong. You should consider all evidence and be open to the reality that we often don't know what we don't know.

It follows that a key aspect of scientific communication and discussion is openness and understanding that what may be a crazy idea one day may be a vital breakthrough another day. Sydney Brenner was known for his acceptance of ideas that push the boundary of understanding. One of his PhD students said "Sydney would pour out all sorts of rubbish, all sorts of crazy ideas. It was almost as though he was on LSD or something. But he wasn't. They were all bits of crazy making crazy connections."⁵ Perhaps his openness to imaginative thought helped him with his discoveries,

---

* Galileo is said to have uttered this phrase after his condemnation by the Roman Catholic Inquisition of 1633. He was referring to the movement of the Earth and all the planets around the Sun.

which gave him the 2002 Nobel Prize in Physiology or Medicine (shared with Robert Horvitz and John Sulston). Also, five of his students went on to win Nobel Prizes.

Paradigms filter our perception to fit into the prevailing view. It is necessary to pay attention to the influence of our paradigms on our perceptions and on our imagination.

> I like science because when you think of something you can check it by experiment: "Yes" or "No" nature says, and you go on from there progressively. Other wisdom has no equally certain way of separating truth from falsehood.[6]
> —Attributed to Richard Feynman (1918–1988), American theoretical physicist, winner of the 1965 Nobel Prize in Physics

> Do not be too timid and squeamish about your actions. All life is an experiment. The more experiments you make the better. What if they are a little coarse and you may get your coat soiled or torn? What if you do fail and get fairly rolled in the dirt once or twice? Up again, you shall never be so afraid of a tumble.[7]
> —Ralph Waldo Emerson

References

1. Feyerabend P. *Against Method*. Verso; 2020.
2. Einstein A. On the method of theoretical physics. Lecture delivered at Oxford University, June 10, 1933. *Philosophy Sci*. 1934;1(2):163–9.
3. Brenner S, as told to Louis Wolpert. *My Life in Science*. BMC Biomedcentral; 1994.
4. Conniff R. When continental drift was considered pseudoscience. *Smithsonian*. Oct 2012. https://www.smithsonianmag.com/science-nature/when-continental-drift-was-considered-pseudoscience-90353214.
5. Kenyon C. Sydney Brenner (1927–2019). *Science*. 2019 May 17;364(6441):638. doi:10.1126/science.aax8563. PMID: 31097656.
6. Feynman M, Ed., the quotable Feynman, p 81. Princeton University Press; 2015.
7. Emerson RW. *Self Reliance*. Monroe and Co.; 1841.

Lesson 81
There Is Only One Kind of Science, and That Is the Study of Everything with All Possible Methods

The names we have for the disciplines are tools which are imperfect representations of reality. Although they are useful to some degree, they are all artificial. Consider the difference between anatomy and physiology. Clearly a structure which does not exist has no physiology—so anatomy is needed to have physiology. And why would someone want to study the anatomy of an organ without considering its functions?

Where exactly is the border between neurology and psychiatry? If schizophrenia, which is classified as a psychiatric condition, is a behavioral disorder it must be a brain disease. Is neurology not the study of the brain which is responsible for behavior? Epilepsy, which is a brain disease, is handled by neurologists and has many psychological aspects. Is Creutzfeldt-Jakob disease a genetic, degenerative, or infectious condition? (It is all of them.) Is Alzheimer's disease a neurological or a psychiatric condition? Patients with the disease often suffer from depression as well as delusions, hallucinations, and behavioral abnormalities in addition to memory loss. And should Alzheimer's disease be studied by neurologists or geriatricians?

In the 1980s, when I worked at the National Institute on Aging (NIA) of the US National Institutes of Health (NIH) in Bethesda, Maryland, I witnessed a discussion between my lab chief and the institute director. My lab chief complained that the NIH institute devoted to neurology, the National Institute of Neurological Disorders and Stroke (NINDS), had begun to perform research on Alzheimer's disease. He wanted the director to do something to stop the NINDS from working on Alzheimer's because he thought that work on that disease should be restricted to his laboratory in the NIA. I was astounded by his attempt to limit the research of other scientists on an important problem.

We must realize that the disciplines are illusory and the remains of irrational historical developments. A twenty-first-century scientist should not be limited in her explorations by considerations of discipline. This argument is equally applicable to clinical matters, of course. It turns out that the workings of the brain in health and disease are strongly influenced by the microbes that live in the gut. It is no longer necessary or sufficient for the neurologist or psychiatrist to concern themselves only with neurons. Neuronal function is dependent on a myriad number of factors that are not entirely neurological.

Similarly, it is best to be open to the great variety of techniques available for clinical and research studies. It may very well be that the best approach to an important problem lies in a discipline removed from your own. If that is the case, consider learning it yourself or develop collaborations. All the available methods are there for you to consider. The answer to your scientific problem may lie in another field entirely. You need to be open to the possibilities because the potential for human knowledge has no boundaries.

> I'm a great believer in the power of ignorance. I think you can always know too much. I feel that one of the problems about being an experienced scientist in a particular field is that it can curtail creativity because you know too many reasons why something may not work. So I believe that it's people who come from the outside, who have not entrained into the standard approach, who can see things in a different way who can take the next step.[1]
>
> —Sydney Brenner

> I think that research—with very few exceptions—is really a job for young people, largely because, as I've said before, they have the ignorance that is necessary for it.[1]
>
> —Sydney Brenner

Reference

1. Brenner S. *My Life in Science*. BioMed Central Ltd; 2001.

Lesson 82
It's Good To Be First, but It Is Not Necessary

If you have an idea which has already been proposed or demonstrated, it may be that any contribution you may make in regard to your idea will be a valuable confirmation of the earlier work. It may also be important if you fail to replicate the work of others. You may also take your idea and pursue it in a novel way which may be of great importance. Do not assume that your ideas are not worthwhile just because they are not completely, absolutely, and perfectly original.

Here are some famous examples of important contributions which were not completely original.

Edward Jenner (1749–1823) is credited with the discovery of the smallpox vaccine. However, he was not the first scientist or person to be aware of the connection between cowpox (vaccinia) and smallpox (variola). Immunization with cowpox was described in sixteenth-century Ming Dynasty China, as well as in India and Africa. It was also practiced in the Ottoman Empire. Milkmaids (girls and women who handle cows) already knew, before Jenner, that people who had skin lesions from exposure to cows were protected from smallpox.[1] Although Jenner did certainly make contributions to enhancing the scientific basis of the procedure, he was not the originator of the practice of vaccination.

Alexander Fleming (1881–1955) is considered the discoverer of world's first effective antibiotic. He noted that airborne spores of the fungus *Penicillium* diminished growth of the bacterium *Staphylococcus aureus*. Antibacterial features of fungi were previously known in ancient China. However, Fleming's *Penicillium* was superior. He was also not responsible for the development of drugs from his research, which was begun by Ernest Chain and Howard Florey, who won the 1945 Nobel Prize in Physiology or Medicine with Fleming for "the discovery of penicillin and its curative effect on various infectious diseases." A 2007 review of Fleming's discovery is entitled "One sometimes finds what one is not looking for, the most important discovery of the twentieth century (Sir Alexander Fleming)."[2]

Stanley Prusiner coined the term "prion," a proteinaceous infectious agent which lacked nucleic acid, in a paper in *Science* in 1982. He was successful in isolating the prion protein and sequencing it. His lab completed a remarkable series of comprehensive studies to demonstrate the basic principles of prion diseases of humans, which include kuru, Creutzfeldt-Jakob disease, bovine spongiform encephalopathy (mad cow disease), and others. Prusiner was not the first to show that the infectious agent in these disorders had no nucleic acid, and he was not the first to suggest that the infectious agent was a protein. He won the 1999 Nobel Prize in Physiology or Medicine for his contributions.[3]

In 1962, Austrian biochemist Oleh Hornykiewicz (1926–2020) showed that the basal ganglia of patients with Parkinson's disease was deficient in the neurotransmitter dopamine. It was apparent that the opportunity existed for the treatment of the disease with the amino acid precursor of dopamine, dihydroxyphenylalanine (DOPA). Several groups tried to treat patients with Parkinson's disease with oral doses of levodopa and found marked side effects. In 1972, George Cotzias, working at the Brookhaven National Labs, added a L-peripheral dopa decarboxylase inhibitor to decrease the side effects and increased the dose of levodopa.[4] These changes in therapy produced a powerful effect which has great value in the treatment of the disease. Cotzias was not the first to use levodopa for Parkinson's disease, but he found the best dose and made one of the greatest discoveries of twentieth-century neuroscience.

The idea that *Helicobacter pylori* was a cause of peptic ulcer was introduced in 1983. Previously it had been suggested that bacteria were involved in the disease in 1875, and antibiotic treatment for ulcers had been recommended in 1948. This approach was ignored for more than 100 years. Barry Marshall and Robin Warren received the 2005 Nobel Prize in Physiology or Medicine for their "discovery of the bacterium *Helicobacter pylori* and its role in gastritis and peptic ulcer disease."[5]

> In science the credit goes to the man who convinces the world, not to the man to whom the idea first occurs.[6]
> —Francis Darwin, botanist; son of Charles Darwin

> Being first is nice but being correct is more important.
> —Attributed to Philip McHugh

Alexander Fleming (1881–1955): A Person to Know

Fleming was a Scottish physician and microbiologist. In 1928, he noted that growth of mold on a plate of *Staphylococci* destroyed the bacteria. He gave the fungus the name "penicillin." His discovery received little attention at first, and he was not believed. He also discovered lysozymes, compounds produced by the body which inhibit bacterial growth. Fleming received the 1945 Nobel Prize in Physiology or Medicine (jointly with Ernst Boris Chain and Sir Howard Walter Florey) for the discovery of penicillin.

George Cotzias (1918–1977): A Person to Know

Cotzias was a Greek scientist and neurologist. He followed the work of Swedish scientist Arvid Carlson and Polish Oleh Hornykiewicz (1926–2020), who showed that dopamine was a key neurotransmitter involved in basal ganglia pathways controlling movement functions. Cotzias knew that L-dihydroxyphenylalanine (L-dopa, also known as levodopa) was a precursor of dopamine, and he showed, in 1968, that high doses of L-dopa were an effective symptomatic therapy for Parkinson's disease.

References

1. Carrell JL. *The Speckled Monster: A Historical Tale of Battling Smallpox*. Dutton; 2003.
2. Wennergren G, Lagercrantz H. "One sometimes finds what one is not looking for" (Sir Alexander Fleming): The most important medical discovery of the 20th century. *Acta Paediatr*. 2007 Jan;96(1):141–4. doi:10.1111/j.1651-2227.2007.00098.x. PMID: 17187625.
3. Prusiner SB. Novel proteinaceous infectious particles cause scrapie. *Science*. 1982 Apr 9;216(4542):136–44. doi:10.1126/science.6801762. PMID: 6801762.
4. Cotzias GC, Van Woert MH, Schiffer LM. Aromatic amino acids and modification of parkinsonism. *N Engl J Med*. 1967 Feb 16;276(7):374–9. doi:10.1056/NEJM196702162760703. PMID: 5334614
5. Nobel Prize Organization. Barry Marshall Nobel lecture. 2005. https://www.nobelprize.org/prizes/medicine/2005/marshall/lecture/.
6. Darwin D. *Eugenics Review*. April 1914.

Lesson 83
You Don't Need To Be Brilliant To Be a Researcher

People who are identified as being extremely intelligent are often those who have either outstanding memory or great verbal skills, or both. Having an outstanding memory and great verbal skills are powerful aids to success in school and university. It does not always translate that such individuals make great doctors or scientists, however. One professor of mine during my residency could remember his patient's previous admissions going back several decades, including which bed they had occupied. We found this ability very impressive at the time, but in retrospect it is meaningless. Many renowned persons in medicine do not have great verbal skills or great memory abilities. What is important for success in medicine and science is imagination and perseverance.

Persons who are identified as extremely intelligent may do well in school without working hard. Once they graduate and start their practice of medicine or science they will not succeed without hard work. Do not allow your imagination and ambition to be limited by what you perceive to be your intellectual shortcomings.

There is a story told by Buddhist author Jack Kornfield about a woman who was depressed after surgery for breast cancer. She was a singer who believed that her career was over following surgery. In the hospital, she was introduced to a volunteer who had had one leg removed because of cancer. He showed her how he could still dance. She said to him "If you can dance, I can sing."[1] Similarly, I see it as the responsibly of physicians at all levels of academic accomplishment to contribute to the global effort to understand disease.

Mathematics is a very important part of science and medicine. If you're good in math that's terrific; it may be very helpful in your career. If you're not good in math, it will not be an impediment in many fields. Advanced math is crucial for astrophysics but is not necessary for cardiology, neurology, or microbiology, for example. Positron emission tomography involves complex math for the reconstruction of the image from the data collected from the detectors. This math has already been accomplished, and it is not necessary for persons using the technique to understand it. Entomologist Edward Wilson emphasizes the point that mathematical expertise is not needed for scientific accomplishment in his *Letters to a Young Scientist*.[2] He says, "mathematical fluency is not enough."

Canadian architect Frank Gehry is widely admired for his innovative design of buildings in the United States, Spain, France, and elsewhere. He designs his work by making architectural models from torn paper, glue, tape, cardboard, apples, and water bottles. He does not himself know how to use a computer. He contributes the ideas, and it is left to others to apply them to the work. Advanced competence with computer languages and capacities is highly desirable to medicine and science. But it is not absolutory necessary.

> [S]uccessful research doesn't depend on mathematical skill, or even the deep understanding of theory. It depends to a large degree on choosing an important problem and finding a way to solve it, even if imperfectly at first. Very often ambition and entrepreneurial drive, in combination, beat brilliance.[2]
>
> —Edward O. Wilson

> There are no rules of logic for making discoveries, let alone for converting those lacking in natural talent for thinking logically into successful researchers.... Discoveries are not the fruit of outstanding talent, but rather of common sense enhanced and strengthened by technical education and the habit of thinking about scientific problems. Thus, anyone with mental gifts balanced enough to cope with everyday life may use them to progress successfully along the road of investigation.
>
> —Santiago Ramon y Cajal[3]

References

1. Kornfield J. *A Path with Heart: A Guide Through the Perils and Promises of a Spiritual Life*. Bantam; 1993.
2. Wilson EO. *Letters to Young Scientists*. Norton; 2013.
3. Ramon y Cajal S. *Cerebrum* 2016 Sep-Oct:11–16.

Lesson 84
Appreciate a Diversity of Approaches

It is beneficial to approach scientific questions using a variety of methods. Studies of humans, animals, organoids, cells, and molecules may all be helpful.* The use of animals in research needs to be informed by an understanding of how the animal is different from the human condition and what is the goal of the project. Mice are very valuable for research but they are not little humans in white fur suits. Fruit flies (*Drosophila*) have proved to be valuable tools for research (particularly because of their short lifespan, relatively low expense, and availability of genetic models), and they have been involved in six Nobel Prizes. If you are studying hair follicles, it may not be wise to involve chickens because they do not have hair. If you are studying the effect of a mutation on gene expression, *Drosophila* may be a good choice.

Nobel Prize–winning pharmacologist Albert Szent-Györgyi believed that humans, animals, cells, and molecules were all to complex, which led him to study the nucleus of the atom as a key factor in cancer. His pursuit of oversimplification was not successful.

Many animal studies are done as basic science without consideration of human disorders. It is worthwhile to consider that the main research funding source in the United States is the National Institutes of Health (NIH) and not the National Institute of Mouse Biology (NIMB).

I had a coworker who had a NIH grant proposal rejected with the reviewer's comment that "the human frontal lobe is too complex to study." The frontal lobe is the largest of our four lobes of cortex and the most evolutionarily recent development. It certainly is complex. What's interesting about this quote is that the complexity of the human frontal lobe cannot be studied in animals because all non-human animals do not have an equivalently complex frontal lobe! Certainly, aspects of cortical function can be studied in animals but there are aspects of our cortical function which cannot be found in nonhuman primates. It is unreasonable to assume that all studies of human frontal lobes are not worthwhile.

Microbiologist and humanist Rene Dubos supported the scientific justification of studies of humans. "In my opinion ... it is unjustified, as well as a defeatist attitude, to pretend that the experiential complexities of living man cannot be studied scientifically, until his submicroscopic constituents and elementary reactions have been fully elucidated. Just as the performance of an electronic computer can be described

---

* Organoids are miniaturized versions of organs produced in vitro.

without familiarity with the chemical composition of its wiring and housing, so can useful knowledge of the organism's responses be gained without full understanding of the makeup and operations of its sub microscopic parts.[1,†]

Model systems are often extensively tested and then established and widely used. Assumptions involved in the models are often lost with time. This can lead to errors in technical matters as well as in interpretation of data.

In 2011, a team of researchers reported in a major international journal the results of a study of the effects of aging on the electrophysiology of the brain in Rhesus monkeys. The results were interpreted as showing which changes in the brain are responsible for age-related cognitive decline. A colleague of mine, Changiz Geula of Northwestern University, and I wrote a letter to the editors of the journal pointing out that the monkeys studied had experienced years of physical and emotional deprivation because they lived in an animal facility and not in a natural environment. We suggested that the possibility that the observed changes in the brain were caused by this potent environmental factor should be addressed in the paper. The authors responded that our remarks would damage public attitudes concerning the use of monkeys in research. They stated that because the monkeys had their needs met and did not have to fight for their food, as they would have in the wilderness, they were "more like humans." They also said that because the cognitive changes in the monkeys were similar to what happens in humans that these changes were not caused by captivity.

It is fundamental that animal research be presented and discussed honestly and openly. It is obvious that a lifetime of social isolation will have effects on the brain. In addition, the observation that the decline of cognition in the monkeys was similar to that in humans cannot be used as evidence that the decline in the monkeys was *not* caused by social isolation. This is a logical fallacy (an argument which sounds convincing but is actually flawed). A key factor of the research was to observe cognitive decline with age. Did the authors consider the possibility that cognition did not decline with age in the monkeys but was observed to decline only because of social isolation? It is desirable that monkeys used in studies have the richest possible mental and social life. However, the actual nature of their life experience, in comparison to their natural environment, needs to be recognized.[‡]

I heard an excellent talk one day about the neurophysiology of the visual system in the thalamus of mice. I asked the speaker if he had considered the fact that humans are visual creatures, as 85% of the input through our brains comes from vision. Mice, on the other hand, are primarily olfactory. Would this difference in function affect the ability to learn about human vision from studies of mouse vision? And could he tell me what were the implications of his work in mouse models for understanding vision in humans? I was disturbed that he had not thought of how to address my question and that the question had never occurred to him. The story of the man looking for

---

[†] Dubos wrote an excellent scientific biography of Louis Pasteur.[2]
[‡] Details about this paper are not included because of the need for confidentiality.

his keys under the lamppost comes to mind. It is certainly reasonable to study vision in mice, but it is necessary to consider what will be learned that may be of interest for human function and disease.

The issue of diversity is also important in clinical matters. Often, the key to diagnosis and treatment can be found only after completion of studies involving biochemistry, histology, immunology, neuroimaging, and other approaches. It is critical that the diverse methods that are applied are all based on the patient's problems. That is, tests should be done only when the information they provide will help patient management.

> Seek diversity to solve complexity.[3]
> —Katrin Prager, Scottish social scientist

> Don't blind yourself and your teammates to potential solutions that could elude you, just because the entire team thinks and approaches problems in the same way. Seek the broadest variety of team members that you can find. A wide range of perspectives brings unique insight.
> —Katrin Prager, Scottish social scientist

Albert Szent-Györgyi (1893–1986): A Person to Know

Hungarian biochemist and winner of the 1937 Nobel Prize in Physiology or Medicine for isolating vitamin C, Szent-Györgyi also helped elucidate the details of the citric acid cycle and uncovered the roles of actin, myosin, and ATP in muscle fibers. He was among the first to study free radicals as a cause of cancer. He said "A discovery must be, by definition, at variance with existing knowledge."[4] His autobiographical essay, *Lost in the 20th Century*, describes his search for diversity of experimental approaches.[5]

References

1. Dubos R. *Man Adapting*. Yale University Press; 1965: xix.
2. Dubos R. *Louis Pasteur: Free Lance of Science*. Da Capo Press; 1986.
3. Prager K. Seek diversity to solve complexity. *Nature*. 2021. PMID: 34211172.
4. Szent-Györgyi A. Dionysians and apollonians. *Science*. 1972 Jun 2;176(4038):966. doi:10.1126/science.176.4038.966. PMID: 17778411.
5. Szent-Györgyi A. Lost in the 20th century. *Ann Rev Biochem*. 1963;32:1–15.

Lesson 85
Why Think When You Can Experiment?

> Why think when you can experiment? Exhaust experiment and then think.[1]
>
> —Claude Bernard

The great French physiologist Claude Bernard (1813–1878), whom we met in Lesson 14, appreciated the value of experimentation and the danger of excessive contemplation. He knew that thought can *guide* experimentation, but he did not want thought to *replace* experimentation. In his 1876 book, *An Introduction to Experimental Medicine* (available from Dover Press in an English translation[1]), he shows how experimental work often taught him that his leading thoughts concerning a problem were mistaken. When this happened, he said he was glad because he had learned something.

Sir Francis Bacon tells a story of a meeting of Catholic monks in the Middle Ages, when the monks were discussing how many teeth were present in the mouth of the horse. One young monk suggested that the answer could be found by going outside, looking inside the horse's mouth, and counting. Reportedly the young monk was expelled from the meeting.

The idea that experimentation can be more important than thinking has many applications to clinical medicine. If you were wondering whether a clinical syndrome could be caused by vitamin B_{12} deficiency, it is clearly indicated to quickly measure the B_{12} level. If your patient fell down the stairs and has weakness and sensory loss in the legs, you should certainly proceed urgently to evaluate the spine with X-rays and MRI. (Do not spend hours on the history and exam.)

The possible danger of excessive thinking can be related to advice about reading. Nobel Prize–winning immunologist Peter Medawar advised against excessive reading and suggested investigation instead. Co-discoverer of the structure of DNA and another Nobel laureate, Francis Crick wrote in large letters on the wall behind his desk "reading rusts the mind." When I was a neurology resident, I was asked by my department chair to write up a case he had of an adolescent girl with chorea coming from mononucleosis.[2] (*Chorea* is an involuntary sudden movement of the arms, leg, or face.) My chair told me that it had never been previously reported as a complication of mononucleosis (an infection with the Epstein-Barr virus). As a young student of neurology eager to learn, I immersed myself in the literature reading every paper ever written about mononucleosis and the brain. I found a paper from 1970, in French, which described patients with chorea as a complication of mononucleosis.

I was proud of my discovery but disappointed to see that my Chair was upset because I had proved him to be in error. He refused to submit the paper for publication for a year.

It is not necessary to know everything about a subject before you investigate. It is desirable to find the middle road. That is, learn enough to know what is happening without exhausting yourself. This is especially true today because the literature is expanding at an incredible rate and no one is able to read all the papers that are possibly relevant to any scientific enterprise.*

Do not let the ideal experiment stop you from doing a good experiment. Remember how limited were the resources of Louis Pasteur in Paris or Frederick Banting in Toronto (Lessons 6 and 88).

Consider what resources may be available. Through collaboration you may vastly improve the speed by which an experiment can be completed (Lesson 71). Currently several international consortia have collected data about conditions such as Alzheimer's disease, Parkinson's disease, cancer, and many others. Collaborations can be developed that are based on use of tissue or other materials which are already available. There may also be data available in these consortium databases about risk factors, socioeconomic aspects, and other features. Often access can be made available to materials and data after a review process.

Another way to proceed rapidly to experimentation is to include yourself as a research participant. Barry Marshall performed a critical experiment on himself demonstrating the ability of *Helicobacter pylori* to cause peptic ulcer disease (Lessons 73 and 85). Pharmacologist Albert Hoffman discovered the psychedelic effects of lysergic acid diethylamide (LSD) through self-experimentation. The appropriately named British neurologist Henry Head helped to define the nerve distribution in his left hand by having a peripheral nerves severed.†

Mauritian neurologist Charles-Eduard Brown-Sequard injected himself with a solution of testicles from dogs and guinea pigs. He claimed that his preparation was an effective treatment for aging, dorsalis (syphilis), tuberculosis, and Parkinson's disease. His method was widely adapted throughout the world (called organotherapy), even though it was dangerous and ineffective. The method served to discredit the field of endocrinology, which was just beginning, and may have delayed the discovery of insulin. Organotherapy was popular because it made physicians and chemists wealthy. It was said that "his ideas were ahead of his time while his method was far behind."[3] Brown Sequard and Claude Bernard (Lesson 47) have jointly been credited with developing the doctrine of internal secretions, which is the foundation of endocrinology.

---

* Recently I learned of an important immune response gene and protein called MYD88 (Innate Immune Signal Transduction Adaptor). I looked it up in the National Library of Medicine database and found that there were 10,875 papers about the molecule (as of August 2023). My lifespan will not be long enough time to read all those papers.

† The description of Dr. Head's work was published in 1961, in the journal *Brain*, by its editor, Russell Brain. (No, I'm not making this up.)

The head of the laboratory where I worked at the University of California, Berkeley, was biophysicist Thomas Budinger, who helped to establish positron emission tomography (PET) methodology. He did arterial catheterization studies on himself to evaluate the important PET input function and made many other important contributions to imaging science.

These examples are not provided to suggest that you try self-experimentation, but rather to point out ways in which doctors and scientists have found novel avenues for exploration.

Doctors have also produced important work in describing their own illnesses. Neuroanatomist Jill Bolte Taylor described her severe stroke in a TED talk.[4] Norwegian professor of medicine Alf Brodal reported his self-observations and neuroanatomical considerations after a stroke with left hemiparesis. British neurologist Oliver Sacks has provided a compelling story about his own responses to injury, in which he felt that his injured leg was no longer a part of his body.[5]

Think also about what data and materials can be found locally. I had a ganglion cyst in my knee which was drained by a hand surgeon. Ganglion cysts are small fluid-filled cavities that grow near a joint. I asked my orthopedist what was the cause of the cyst, and he told me that he didn't know—this as he withdrew several cc's of fluid from my cyst. I wondered what was happening to the cytokines and immune cells in the material he was collecting, which he was about to discard (cytokines are signaling proteins that influence inflammation).

Stroke is the leading cause of disability worldwide. It is widely appreciated that stroke has an important immunological component.[6] Interventional neurologists, neurosurgeons, and neuroradiologists have developed techniques in which clots can be removed from vessels acutely to relieve ischemia. This precious material is routinely discarded or sent to the pathologist, who will likely record it as a thrombus (a clot). The thrombus removed from a clotted blood vessel should be studied for immune proteins, clotting factors, immune cells, and viral and bacterial DNA as well as other things. However, it is routinely discarded (Lesson 93).

Similarly, the tonsils are lymph nodes in the back of the mouth and top of the throat. They are routinely removed because of repeated infections in children and adults. They could be used for valuable studies of immune processes involving drainage of proteins from the brain via newly discovered pathways.[7]

> The "do not think but try" attitude of mind is the important one to cultivate.
> —Attributed to **John Hunter (1728–1793)** Scottish surgeon

> The best way to prepare for an heroic voyage in science is just start.[10]
> —Sydney Brenner

Francis Crick (1916–2004): A Person to Know

Crick was an English molecular biologists and a neuroscientist. Together with James Watson and Maurice Wilkins he won the 1962 Nobel Prize "for their discoveries concerning the molecular structure of nucleic acids and its significance for information transfer in living material" [8]. He clarified the pathways of information transmission from DNA to RNA to protein. His early work was in physics, and, at 31 years of age, he moved to biology, along with several other physicists. Later in life he became interested in neuroscience and the central question of the origin of consciousness. His moves from physics to molecular biology to consciousness are described in his book, *What Mad Pursuit: A Personal View of Scientific Discovery*.[10]

References

1. Bernard C. *An Introduction to the Study of Experimental Medicine*. Dover Books; 1927.
2. Friedland R, Yahr MD. Meningoencephalopathy secondary to infectious mononucleosis: Unusual presentation with stupor and chorea. *Arch Neurol*. 1977 Mar;34(3):186–8. doi:10.1001/archneur.1977.00500150072014. PMID: 190986.
3. Tattersall RB. Charles-Edouard Brown-Sequard, double hyphenated neurologist and forgotten father of endocrinology. *Diabetic Med*. 1994;11: 720–31.
4. Bolte Taylor J. *My Stroke of Insight*. Penguin; 2009.
5. Sacks O. *A Leg to Stand On*. Touchstone; 1984.
6. Tonomura S, Ihara M, Friedland RP. Microbiota in cerebrovascular disease: A key player and future therapeutic target. *J Cereb Blood Flow Metab*. 2020 Jul;40(7):1368–80. doi:10.1177/0271678X20918031. Epub 2020 Apr 20. PMID: 32312168; PMCID: PMC7308516.
7. Rustenhoven J, Kipnis J. Brain borders at the central stage of neuroimmunology. *Nature*. 2022 Dec;612(7940):417–29. doi:10.1038/s41586-022-05474-7. Epub 2022 Dec 14. PMID: 36517712; PMCID: PMC10205171.
8. The Nobel Prize in Physiology or Medicine 1962. Nobel Prize Site for Nobel Prize in Physiology or Medicine 1962.
9. Crick F. *What Mad Pursuit: A Personal View of Scientific Discovery*. Basic Books; 1988.
10. Brenner S. *My Life in Science*; 2001: 0954027809.

Lesson 86
Judge Every Project by Asking "What Difference Will It Make To Know the Answer?"

There have been times when I've wondered if the main motivating feature of scientific investigations was like that of a mountaineer. When the British climber George Mallory was asked by a journalist why he wanted to climb Mount Everest, he reportedly said, "because it's there." (He died on Everest in 1924.) Often it is clear that a new tool was applied to an old problem because the new tool was available and it hadn't been done before. Similarly, in clinical medicine, laboratory and imaging tests are often done because they can be, not because they're indicated. Sometimes the additional tests are poorly justified with the rationale that they are helpful for "completeness."

Another aspect of the choice of methods of investigation is best illustrated by the old story of the man looking for his keys at night under the lamppost. A policeman sees a man looking at the ground under a streetlight at night and asks, "What are you looking for?" The man says, "I lost my keys." They both look on the ground for a while before the policeman asks if he's certain that he lost his keys here, and the man says "No." The policeman asks "Why are you looking for them here?" And the man says, "Because this is where the light is." It is worthwhile to be sure that clinical and investigative approaches are not selected because they are available even though they are not indicated.

It is valuable to always ask these two questions concerning clinical or research investigations: (1) What do you want to learn? And (2), What difference will it make to know the answer?

Unnecessary lab tests and imaging can produce excessive costs and also hazards. Many years ago I heard of a medical student who volunteered to have an electroencephalograph (EEG) taken to teach a group of students on a neurology clerkship. The EEG showed an abnormality that was followed-up with a cerebral angiogram, which caused a stroke. It is well-recognized that unnecessary imaging tests can find unexpected abnormalities called "incidentalomas."[1] Investigation of these unexpected findings involves significant risk.

In one laboratory I worked in, the lab chief liked to do research only when he knew the answer in advance. He proposed a project with enormous expenses and administration of radiation to human participants. I protested because I thought the project was trivial. I knew what the answer would be, and I knew that it would not be significant. He told me "I don't care if it's trivial, I just want to know that it can be published." This is not an uncommon attitude, and is supported by scientific journals that have specific guidelines saying that research significance should not be judged.

According to the *Nature* journal *Scientific Reports* "To be published ... a paper must be scientifically valid and technically sound in methodology and analysis. Manuscripts are not assessed based on their perceived importance, significance or impact; the research community makes such judgements after publication."[2] I am concerned that this position encourages completion of investigations of little impact. *Scientific Reports* publishes more than 22,000 papers every year (National Library of Medicine).

It is true, of course, that surprising findings can have significant unforeseen impact. The history of science is filled with stories about apparently trivial projects leading to great discoveries. If we had greater resources, we would welcome the pursuit of all questions without preconceived ideas. However, our patients need help now, and we should use available resources to pursue the answers we need as best we can.

> To yield to every whim of curiosity, and to allow our passion for inquiry to be restrained by nothing but the limits of our ability, this shows an eagerness of mind not unbecoming to scholarship. But it is wisdom that has the merit of selecting from among the innumerable problems which present themselves, those whose solution is important to mankind.[3]
> —Immanuel Kant, German philosopher (1724–1804)

References

1. Sconfienza E, Tetti M, Forestiero V, Veglio F, Mulatero P, Monticone S. Prevalence of functioning adrenal incidentalomas: A systematic review and meta-analysis. *J Clin Endocrinol Metab*. 2023 Jan 31:dgad044. doi:10.1210/clinem/dgad044. Epub ahead of print. PMID: 36718682.
2. https://www.nature.com/srep/guide-to-referees. Accessed August 26, 2024.
3. Hazlitt H. *The Wisdom of Henry Hazlitt*; Chapter 5, 1993.

Lesson 87
What Is Important in Research

> "What is important in research is whether it is fundamental or trivial, good or bad."
>
> —Alvan Feinstein[1]

The dichotomy between the basic and applied sciences is not useful. To do basic science, do you need to be sure there is no application? And is it not possible to make fundamental discoveries about the natural world when doing applied sciences? If basic science is what is done purely for its own sake (*because it is there*) does that mean that mountaineering is basic science?[1] **What is important in research is whether it is good or bad, not basic or applied, experimental or observational.**

Louis Pasteur's contributions had many practical applications, including anthrax, cholera, and rabies vaccines; the understanding that fermentation is a biological process; treatment of silkworm disease; pasteurization; and understanding of stereochemistry. He did not consider his work to be applied science, as he said, "There are no applied sciences ... there are only ... the applications of science, and this is a very different matter."

A founder of the field of clinical epidemiology, Alvan Feinstein said that there was no such thing as basic science because "Every aspect of human knowledge is constantly, inevitably basic to something and applied from something else."

It is wrong to conclude that clinical research is not important because it is not basic science. As explained by Feinstein, the "basic particle" in physiology is an organ system, in biochemistry a molecule, in philosophy an idea. And the basic particle in clinical medicine is a sick person. The clear goal in clinical medicine is to prevent and treat disease and to provide comfort. This requires understanding at all levels.

The physician has an advantage over the basic scientist because of her experience with patients. Clinical experience is the key factor in illuminating the researcher about what is important. Nonclinicians can attend lectures and read books and articles that do not provide an experiential background equivalent to that of a clinician. At the same time, of course, the clinical investigator may not have knowledge equivalent to a basic scientist about the fine details of disease processes at a molecular level.

The two key words in this matter are *diversity* and *collaboration*. Disease investigations should consider molecular issues as well as systemic matters involving the patient. Collaboration between clinicians and basic scientists is critical for the accomplishment of progress (Lesson 71).

What makes it science is the effectiveness, not the type, of methods used by the investigator. What makes it fundamental is the type of goal it seeks, not the absence of a purpose; and how it is done, not where it is done. What makes it good is the way the investigator uses his artistic imagination and his intellectual discipline to choose problems, ask questions, design plans, execute procedures, analyze data, draw conclusions, and communicate results.

—Alvan Feinstein[1]

Reference

1. Feinstein A. *Clinical Judgment*. Williams and Wilkins; 1967: 390.

Lesson 88
Do Not Be Obsessed with Technology and Methods

The British physician James Parkinson provided the first description of the disease for which he is known in 1817 solely through observation and attention to detail.[1] He did not have access to neuroimaging, cerebrospinal fluid (CSF) analysis, electrophysiology, or postmortem examinations. His work has been widely praised for its clarity and accuracy.*

The great French neurologist Jean-Martin Charcot noted that Parkinson's greatest ability was his powers of observation.[2] He remarked: "Let someone say of a doctor that she really knows her physiology or anatomy.... These are not real compliments; but, if you say she is an observer, a person who knows how to see, this is perhaps the greatest compliment one can make." It was Charcot who suggested that the condition be named after James Parkinson.

In 1890, Charles S. Roy and Charles S. Sherrington published a paper "On the regulation of the blood-supply of the brain" in the *Journal of Physiology*, London.[3] The report made the important conclusion that "The blood supply of any part of the cerebral tissue is varied in accordance with the activity of the chemical changes which underlie the functional action of that part. Bearing in mind that strong evidence exists of localization of function in the brain, we are of opinion that an automatic mechanism, of the kind just referred to, is well fitted to provide for a local variation of the blood-supply in accordance with local variations of the functional activity." This conclusion involved a brilliant series of deductions which describes crucial relationships among blood flow, metabolism, and activity in the brain that was only verified by experiments performed nearly 100 years later. The methods used by Roy and Sherrington involved opening the skull of anesthetized dogs and recording changes in the surface pressure of the brain using a recording apparatus called an oncograph. CSF was permitted to escape freely. The effect of many factors was studied, including the influence of intracarotid administration of filtered brain extracts from the cerebral hemispheres of dogs that had been exsanguinated with the heads kept in an incubator for 4 hours at 37° C.

There are countless additional examples where a great work has been done with primitive measures. Great science often does not require advanced technology.

---

* His short description of the disease is a classic and is available.[1]

Frederick Banting and Charles Best are credited with the discovery of insulin.[4] Banting, the son of a farmer, worked under the direction of John Macleod at the University of Toronto. He had no research experience, no publications, no doctorate, and was initially working without pay. He was assisted by a medical student, Charles Best. They had to buy dogs on the street for research and had a small laboratory. Early on Banting could not even spell the word "diabetes." Banting and Best showed that removal of the dog's pancreas caused diabetes, which could be successfully treated with a pancreatic extract. In 1923, Banting and John Macleod were awarded the Nobel Prize in Physiology or Medicine for the discovery of insulin. (Macleod was Banting's supervisor.) Banting was 32 when he won the prize and remains the youngest recipient of Nobel Prize in Physiology or Medicine. He shared half of the prize money with Best, and with others sold the patent for insulin to the University of Toronto for $1 because Banting thought that economic gain by physicians was contrary to his Hippocratic Oath.

Although technology is often vital to advances in science, it is usually not as important as the quality of the question being addressed. Technical matters can often be assigned to coworkers. It is critical that investigators understand the strengths, limitations, and assumptions of the techniques which are being applied.

There is also a danger that over dependence on technology can impair the flexibility of your career. If you are 100% devoted to a new technique, you may find it difficult to adapt when that technique becomes replaced by newer methods.

> Success in science comes from people, not equipment.
> —Attributed to Peter Kapitsa (1894–1984),
> Soviet physicist and Nobel laureate

Sir Charles S. Sherrington (1857–1951): A Person to Know

Sherrington was a British neurophysiologist who elucidated many pathways of nervous system functioning, including the spinal reflex and elements of neuronal transmission. He coined the term "synapse," and his work is summarized in his important 1906 work, *The Integrative Action of the Nervous System*. He received the 1932 Nobel Prize in Physiology or Medicine together with Edgar Adrian "for their discoveries regarding the functions of neurons." His Nobel lecture, "Inhibition as a coordinative factor," presented his elegant work on the role of inhibition, excitation, and disinhibition on neural activity (disinhibition refers to a failure of inhibition).

References

1. Parkinson J. An essay on the shaking palsy: Neuropsychiatry classics. *J Neuropsychiatry Clin Neurosci*. 2002;14:2.
2. Lewis C. *The Enlightened Mr. Parkinson*. Pegasus; 2017.
3. Friedland RP, Iadecola CR. Roy and Sherrington (1890): A centennial reexamination of "On the regulation of the blood-supply of the brain." *Neurology*. 1991 Jan;41(1):10–14. doi:10.1212/wnl.41.1.10. PMID: 1985272.
4. Nobel Prize Organization. Frederick Banting Nobel lecture: Diabetes and insulin. Sep 15, 1925. https://www.nobelprize.org/prizes/medicine/1923/banting/lecture/. Accessed Nov 3, 2023.

Lesson 89
Pay Attention to Study Design, Data Analysis, and Statistics

According to the statistician John Tukey, "Far better an approximate answer to the right question, which is often vague, than an exact answer to the wrong question, which can always be made precise."[1]

In the journal *Neuroimage*, in 2009, a group of investigators reported an MRI study of one salmon which was 18 inches long.[2] The fish, which was dead, was shown photographs of people in social situations with particular emotions and asked to determine what emotion the individual showed. Several regions in the brain were shown to be significantly activated by this task. This showed that random noise can yield spurious results even when statistical thresholds such as $P < 0.001$ are used. Multiple comparison corrections are needed (this statistical method counteracts, in part, the problem of multiple testing, decreasing the chance that the results are due to chance alone). If many comparisons are made and the number of participants is small, as in this study of one dead fish, the chances of false-positive findings are great.

It is important to consider both false-negative and false-positive results. False-negative results occur when the data incorrectly indicate that a particular condition is absent. False-positive results, on the other hand, occur when data suggest that a condition is present when it is not. The various forms of bias could contribute to a failure to consider these opportunities for error.

Consider how the data were acquired and whether experimenter bias influenced the results (Lesson 52). Placebo effects may also be involved. The magnitude of placebo effects is directly proportional to the cost, pain, and difficulty of an intervention. This is why traditional remedies often contain bitter spices to make them appear to be powerful. As a moonlighting physician many years ago, I was doing evening house calls in Queens, New York. The manager of the practice had a class on how to complete home visits. He told me that every patient needed to get a vitamin B_{12} injection and that I needed to show each patient the solution I was injecting, which was blue, because it would imply that the medication administered was effective. (I never gave B_{12} shots because they were not indicated.)

If a research study claims to be double-blinded, is that the case? In a placebo controlled double-blind randomized trial the participants as well as the investigators will not be told if the subject is getting the active drug or a placebo. However, the double-blind status only operates if the patient cannot correctly guess which group they are in. This is a quote from a patient in a trial of a medication for amyotrophic lateral sclerosis: "I just had my one month ... trial visit ... today. I am guessing that I am not on placebo because each time I ramped up dosage I was nauseous for 3 days and that's a known side effect." A patient of mine in an Alzheimer's disease treatment trial told me that he was upset that he did not have any side effects in the study. I asked him why, and he said that he assumed that he was not in the active arm since he knew of other participants who were having significant side effects. This is called a *nocebo effect* (the opposite of the placebo effect, a negative outcome occurring due to the belief that the intervention is harmful or not effective).[2]

In one study, the analysis of the effect of treatment with methylene blue on cognition in Alzheimer's disease may have been impaired by the blue discoloration of urine in the group receiving the active agent. This means that the study was no longer double-blinded. In a study of the effect of chelation therapy to remove aluminum from the brain of Alzheimer's disease patients a significant effect was observed, favoring the group receiving the experimental agent.[3] However, the therapy was administered by a painful intramuscular injection, and the comparison treatment was a pill delivered orally.[3] The placebo effect in this case would be enhanced by pain. The investigators claimed that because the main outcome variable was time until death, they thought that the placebo effect could not be involved. However, they failed to consider the response of the caregivers, who would wish to keep the participants alive as long as possible if they thought that they were receiving an active treatment. The power and importance of placebo effect has also been demonstrated in studies using sham surgeries (Lesson 29).

It is prudent not to overinterpret the correlation coefficient as an unequivocal indicator of the strength or weakness of an effect.[4] The correlation coefficient is a measure of the linear correlation between two datasets. The danger of overinterpretation of correlation coefficients is shown by the website Spurious Correlations,[5] which shows highly significant meaningless correlations, such as between the divorce rate in Maine and the per capita consumption of margarine. Significant correlations are also shown between per capita consumption of mozzarella cheese and civil engineering doctorates awarded, and also between the letters in the winning word of the Scripps National Spelling Bee and the number of people killed by venomous spiders.

The first step of data analysis is looking at the data. All the data. Look for things that are obvious.[6] Don't rely only on the summaries, such as the mean and standard deviation, correlation coefficients, and significant or insignificant differences. **Rather than looking at the statistics, look at the data.** In an early PET study of ours in Alzheimer's disease, we found that there was no significant asymmetry of glucose metabolism in a group of participants with the disease (the means were of left and right were the same). Further observation showed us, however, that there was more variability in the Alzheimer's disease group than in the control group because some participants had significantly asymmetrical metabolic defects in the cortex. Some subjects had metabolic defects on the right hemisphere and some had defects in the left, and these asymmetries were related to the behavioral features of the disease.[7] This observation would not have been made if we hadn't looked at the variability in the data.

Francis Dalton, founder of the statistical concept of correlation, expressed a similar thought: "It is difficult to understand why statisticians commonly limit their inquiries to averages, and do not revel in more comprehensive views. Their souls seem as dull to the charm of variety as that of the native of one of our flat English counties, whose retrospect of Switzerland was that, if its mountains could be thrown into its lakes, two nuisances would be got rid of at once."

As implied by John Tukey at the beginning of this lesson and also by the story of the cigar-smoking monks (Epilogue), the critical matter in data analysis and statistics is the question being asked, and how it is asked. The best results are those that are clear without the need for statistics. If data analysis in a clinical trial takes 6 months to complete and involves many statisticians the results should be questioned for fear of data massaging (also referred to as data cleansing and data scrubbing).

If your experiment needs statistics, you ought to have done a better experiment.
—Attributed to Lord Ernest Rutherford, New Zealand physicist (1871–1937)

One man's noise is another man's signal.[8]
—Attributed to Sir Bernard Katz (1911–2003), German British physician, corecipient of the 1970 Nobel Prize in Physiology or Medicine

References

1. Tukey J. *The Future of Data Analysis*. Springer; 1962: 13–14.
2. Bennett CM, Miller MB, Wolford GL. Neural correlates of interspecies perspective taking in the post-mortem Atlantic Salmon: An argument for multiple comparisons correction. *Neuroimage*. 2009; 47(1):S125.
3. Crapper McLachlan DR, Dalton AJ, Kruck TP, Bell MY, Smith WL, Kalow W, Andrews DF. Intramuscular desferrioxamine in patients with Alzheimer's disease. *Lancet*. 1991 Jun 1;337(8753):1304–8. doi:10.1016/0140-6736(91)92978-b. Erratum in: Lancet 1991 Jun 29;337(8757):1618. PMID: 1674295.
4. Rusakov DA. A misadventure of the correlation coefficient. *Trends Neurosci*. 2023 Feb;46(2):94–6. doi:10.1016/j.tins.2022.09.009. Epub 2022 Oct 21. PMID: 36280457.
5. https://www.tylervigen.com/spurious-correlations. Accessed May 22, 2023.
6. Boles RC. Why you should avoid statistics. *Biol Psych*. 1988;23:79–85.
7. Friedland RP, Koss E, Haxby JV, Grady CL, Luxenberg J, Schapiro MB, Kaye J. NIH conference. Alzheimer disease: Clinical and biological heterogeneity. *Ann Intern Med*. 1988 Aug 15;109(4):298–311. doi:10.7326/0003-4819-109-4-298. PMID: 2969203.
8. Friedland RP. Personal communication; 1984.

Lesson 90
Be Aware of (*Beware of*) Statistics and Data Torturing

Statistical analysis can be manipulated to support your preconceived ideas. *Data torturing* is what happens when data are manipulated to prove what the investigator wishes to show. Epidemiologist J. L. Mills suggests there are two kinds of data torturing: one kind is opportunistic, when the data are extensively reviewed until a significant association is found and a biological plausible hypothesis is made to fit.[1] The second, or procrustean form of data torturing, occurs when a hypothesis is chosen and arbitrary data are made to fit it (Procrustes is a thief in Greek mythology who adapted his victims to fit the length of his bed by stretching or cutting off their legs).

Watch out for data torturing: "If you torture your data long enough, they will tell you whatever you want to hear."[1]

Opportunistic data torturers can often get significant results by failing to correct for multiple comparisons. Procrustean data torturing may involve putting research participants into manipulated groups that support the desired outcome. Data can be reanalyzed according to different time intervals. Also, group memberships can be manipulated with suppression of data that are contradictory. Performing multiple analyses until the desired results are obtained can clearly lead to erroneous results.

Biological plausibility may help in analysis of data but may be misleading. When deciding whether the results of a study are likely to be correct, you may consider if there is a biological mechanism to explain the findings. Molecular pathways are so complicated now that it is possible to make anything appear related to anything else.

Remember that statistics may not be necessary if the results are obvious.[2] Penicillin and related antibiotics are effective for pharyngitis caused by group A *Streptococcus*. The profound efficacy of the treatment does not require statistical analysis.

The choice of control groups is often critical. Controls may be matched for gender, age, education, body weight, health status, and many other factors depending on the nature of the project. Be careful and always evaluate whether the controls were properly matched.

Confounding factors must always be considered. For example, if a study investigates the relationship between oral health and stroke, it must also consider the relationship between both oral health and smoking, alcohol abuse, socioeconomic status, education, diet and diabetes. (These factors are also related to stroke.)

Consider "reverse causation." Older persons who are mentally inactive are more likely to develop dementia. It is difficult to distinguish whether this relationship is because low levels of activity accelerate the disease process or because low levels of activity are signs of the disease process itself.[3] Both explanations may be correct.

It is important to look at the data, *all the data*. The summarized data may be important, of course, but there may also be key factors in the variability and raw data (Lesson 89). Important information may be reflected by the outliers.

> If you torture the data long enough, it will confess to anything.[4]
> —Ronald Coase, British economist

References

1. Mills JL. Data torturing. *N Engl J Med*. 1993 Oct 14;329(16):1196–9. doi:10.1056/NEJM199310143291613. PMID: 8166792.
2. Bolles RC. Why you should avoid statistics. *Biol Psychiatry*. 1988 Jan 1;23(1):79–85. doi:10.1016/0006-3223(88)90107-2. PMID: 3337855.
3. Friedland RP, Fritsch T, Smyth KA, Koss E, Lerner AJ, Chen CH, Petot GJ, Debanne SM. Patients with Alzheimer's disease have reduced activities in midlife compared with healthy control-group members. *Proc Natl Acad Sci U S A*. 2001 Mar 13;98(6):3440–5. doi:10.1073/pnas.061002998. Epub 2001 Mar 6. PMID: 11248097; PMCID: PMC30672.
4. Sauvy A. *The Public Option*. Press Universaires de France; 1961: 100.

Lesson 91
Pay Attention to the Assumptions of Diagnostic Testing and Research Evaluations

No diagnostic test or research assay is perfect. Many are excellent and valuable, of course, but they all have limitations. Often these limitations are thoroughly considered when the technology is advanced and then widely forgotten. This failure to consider limitations is often because of the neglect of assumptions. To assume is "to suppose, to take for granted without proof as the basis of argument" (*Oxford English Dictionary*). Certainly, we should be concerned about what ideas or processes we accept without proof.

A good example is the most popular animal model, the mouse. Although it is an outstanding model of human disease, it is not a primate. This is not to say that we cannot learn about human disease by studying mice, just that we must remember that it is a rodent and has many significant differences compared to people. There are countless examples of drugs and procedures that have been shown to be effective in mice but failed in human trials. Rodent researchers must not fail to recall that mice are not people.

A standard test of toxicity is the LD50 (50% lethal dose), which is the dose of a substance that kills half of a group of mice after a specified period. Can we assume that a substance with a very high LD50 in mice is safe for humans to consume? The answer must be no because a compound may be carcinogenic and take a long time to kill the animal. Also, the metabolism and detoxification pathways in the liver, such as cytochrome P450, are different in mice and humans.[1] Most notably of course, the cognitive abilities of mice are much simpler than those of humans, and a drug may damage the brain but not alter the LD50.

Functional MRI (fMRI) is a valuable technique that has led to many advances in the localization of function in the cerebral cortex and other aspects of brain function in health and disease. The technique is based on the magnetic qualities of hemoglobin, which vary depending on the presence or absence of oxygen. And the oxygenation status of hemoglobin is related to regional cerebral blood flow in the brain. Because of these relationships it is possible to learn about patterns of activation of neurons in the cerebral cortex, which is closely related to cerebral blood flow.[2] However, this relationship may be altered when there is disease of the cerebral vessels or the innervation of those vessels. This possibility has not been widely considered in fMRI studies.

Cerebrospinal fluid cytology is a valuable test to look for malignant and immune cells as well as infectious agents. However, if the specimen is not properly handled and rapidly assayed, the cells may be lost in time and a false-negative result may be produced.

An early positron emission tomography (PET) study of cerebral metabolism in Down syndrome suggested that the glucose metabolic rate was increased in the cortex. This finding had potentially important implications for the theory that the disease was caused by excessive neuronal activity (excitotoxicity). Subsequent work showed that the glucose metabolic rate was actually normal in Down syndrome. The results in the earlier study may have been caused by failure to consider that individuals with Down syndrome have smaller heads and thus less attenuation of the radiation coming from the brain.[3]

The corpus callosum is the largest fiber tract in the brain. In 1940, neurophysiologist Warren McCulloch suggested that the only known role of this corpus callosum was "to aid in the transmission of epileptic seizures from one to the other side of the brain." In 1951, psychologist Karl Lashley proposed that its purpose "must be mainly mechanical ... i.e., to keep the hemispheres from sagging." (Perhaps he was joking). The true role of the commissure was not discovered until the work of Roger Sperry and Michael Gazzaniga, who studied monkeys as well as patients, who had had the structure severed for the treatment of intractable epilepsy.[4] They found that cutting the commissure did not change motor abilities or cognitive functioning. However, studies of persons after commissurotomy demonstrated intricacies of cerebral hemispheric specialization. The investigators came to the conclusion that each hemisphere is "indeed a conscious system in its own right, perceiving, thinking, remembering, reasoning, willing, and emoting, all at a characteristically human level, and ... both the left and the right hemisphere may be conscious simultaneously in different, even in mutually conflicting, mental experiences that run along in parallel."[4]

Roger Sperry received the 1981 Nobel Prize in Physiology or Medicine for his work. Since then, many people have forgotten that the hemispheric function of hemispherectomized humans is not the same as that of persons with intact commissures. When I use my right cerebral hemisphere, it is able to quickly know what is happening in my left hemisphere because my commissure is intact. (This is not true for Sperry's research participants, who had had their commissure severed.) This misunderstanding has led to an unscientific corpus of work about excessive lateralization of function in the brain and whether each of us are "left-brained" or "right-brained."

Olfactory dysfunction in Alzheimer's disease is expected in view of the strong involvement of the entorhinal cortex and related areas. (*Entorhinal* means relating to the nose.) Studies of olfaction in the disease have shown deficits on tests requiring the naming of odors. These tests are confounded because reduced naming of odors can be caused by either language disturbance or difficulty with olfactory detection. Linguistic problems, which are common in the disease, can certainly contribute to impaired naming of odors. Odor naming would be expected to be relatively fragile, as naming odors is not something that persons do frequently. A more appropriate assessment of olfaction involves measurement of olfactory threshold, a task without the need of cognitive processing.[5]

It is necessary to understand the scientific background of the technologies that you use in clinical practice and research.

Roger W. Sperry (1913–1994): A Person to Know

Sperry was an American cognitive neuroscientist. While he was a student at Oberlin College, he studied under R. H. Stetson, who was a student of William James. He was denied tenure at the University of Chicago and moved to the California Institute of Technology, where he worked for several decades. Sperry was interested in neural circuits and neuronal specificity. His work was aided by collaboration with neurosurgeon Joseph Bogen, who performed the commissurotomies. He won the 1981 Nobel Prize in Physiology and Medicine with David Hubel and Torsten Wiesel.[6,7]

References

1. Yoshizato K, Tateno C, Utoh R. Mice with liver composed of human hepatocytes as an animal model for drug testing. *Curr Drug Discov Technol.* 2012 Mar;9(1):63–76. doi:10.2174/157016312799304570. PMID: 22023259.
2. Lai S, Hopkins AL, Haacke EM, Li D, Wasserman BA, Buckley P, Friedman L, Meltzer H, Hedera P, Friedland R. Identification of vascular structures as a major source of signal contrast in high resolution 2D and 3D functional activation imaging of the motor cortex at 1.5T: Preliminary results. *Magn Reson Med.* 1993 Sep;30(3):387–92. doi:10.1002/mrm.1910300318. PMID: 8412613.
3. Schapiro MB, Grady CL, Kumar A, Herscovitch P, Haxby JV, Moore AM, White B, Friedland RP, Rapoport SI. Regional cerebral glucose metabolism is normal in young adults with Down syndrome. *J Cereb Blood Flow Metab.* 1990 Mar;10(2):199–206. doi:10.1038/jcbfm.1990.35. PMID: 2137464.
4. Hubel D. Roger W. Sperry (1913–1994). *Nature.* 1994;369(6477):186. Bibcode:1994Natur.369.186H. doi:10.1038/369186a0. PMID 8183336. S2CID 29829822.
5. Koss E, Weiffenbach JM, Haxby JV, Friedland RP. Olfactory detection and identification performance are dissociated in early Alzheimer's disease. *Neurology.* 1988 Aug;38(8):1228–32. doi:10.1212/wnl.38.8.1228. PMID: 3399073.
6. Horowitz NH. *Roger Wolcott Sperry.* Nobel Prize in Physiology or Medicine; 1981.
7. Sperry RW. The great cerebral commissure, *Sci Am.* 1964 Jan;210:42–52. doi:10.1038/scientificamerican0164-42. PMID: 14088562.

Lesson 92
It Is Possible To Be Productive from a Distance

In the 1950s, an epidemic of a new deadly neurological disease called kuru was observed in the Eastern Highlands of New Guinea. Talented and tenacious pediatrician Daniel Carlton Gajdusek was sent by the US National Institutes of Health to investigate. He found that the disease affected primarily children of both sexes and women. Rigorous investigations failed to show that the disease had an infectious, genetic, toxic, traumatic, vascular, or nutritional origin. In 1959, the investigators published the neuropathology of this unique brain degeneration.[1,2]

British veterinary pathologist William Hadlow saw the report and wrote a letter to *The Lancet* in which he pointed out the structural similarity between kuru and a disease of sheep called *scrapie*, which was well known to be transmissible from animal to animal.[3] Hadlow said "While attempts to draw too close in analogy between diseases of man and lower animals are attended by numerous pitfalls, many valuable clues contributing to the understanding of the fundamental nature of a disease can be gained from a broad comparative viewpoint." Gajdusek and colleagues read the letter and tested the transmissibility of kuru by injecting the brains of three chimpanzees with material from kuru patients. They became affected years later, thus demonstrating that kuru could be transmitted by cannibalism, which was practiced in the tribe who suffered from kuru. They also later showed that a rapidly progressive cause of dementia, Creutzfeldt-Jakob disease, is also transmissible from humans to chimps.

Hadlow's letter played a vital role in leading Gajdusek's group to the next stage of their investigations. Gajdusek later denied that Hadlow's letter influenced his work.[4]

In 1979, I published a letter in a scientific journal concerning a rather minor error concerning cerebral blood flow and hematocrit (a measure of what percentage of the blood is taken up by red blood cells). A few months later the editor of the *American Heart Journal* called me and said that since I was an expert on the subject of blood flow and hematocrit, I should write an editorial. I was certainly not an expert, but with the help of a friend who is a hematologist we completed the editorial.[5]

It is a remarkable truth that the scientific literature has a globally diverse audience, and one never knows what will develop following publications, even letters!

Daniel Carleton Gajdusek (1924–2008): A Person to Know

Gajdusek was an born in Yonkers, New York, and worked as a virologist at the Walter Reed Army Medical Service Graduate School. While he was a visiting investigator in Australia he learned of an unusual and novel neurological disease, kuru, in the Highlands of New Guinea. As a laboratory chief at the National Institutes of Health he investigated the condition and showed that it was transmissible to nonhuman primates. For this discovery he was a co-recipient of the 1976 Nobel Prize in Physiology or Medicine.[1,2] (The contribution of the chimpanzees Daisey, Joanne, and Georgette to the research was acknowledged in Gadjusek et al.'s paper published in *Nature*.[1])

References

1. Beck E, Daniel PM, Asher DM, Gajdusek DC, Gibbs CJ Jr. Experimental kuru in the chimpanzee: A neuropathological study. *Brain*. 1973 Sep;96(3):441–62. doi:10.1093/brain/96.3.441. PMID: 4200638.
2. Klatzo I, Gajdusek Dc, Zigas V. Pathology of kuru. *Lab Invest*. 1959 Jul-Aug;8(4):799–847. PMID: 13665963
3. Hadlow WJ. Kuru likened to scrapie: the story remembered. *Philos Trans R Soc Lond B Biol Sci*. 2008 Nov 27;*363*(1510):3644. doi:10.1098/rstb.2008.4013. PMID: 18849258; PMCID: PMC2735530.
4. Carleton Gajdusek D. Personal communication; 1989.
5. Friedland RP, Grant S. Hematocrit, viscosity and cerebral blood flow. *Am Heart J*. 1979;97:404–5. ISSN 0002-8703.

Lesson 93
You Can Make Contributions as a Clinician Without a Laboratory

For most of the past several hundred years great advances in medicine have been provided by doctors based on their experience with patients. In today's highly technological world, in which protein expression patterns from single cells can be measured and genes transferred between organisms and manipulated precisely, it is tempting to think that the day in which great advances are made by practicing physicians is over. This is most definitely not the case. Here are some examples in which practicing physicians have made great discoveries based on their experience with patients.

Irving Cooper was a neurosurgeon practicing at New York University. In 1952, he was operating on the brain of a patient with severe tremor, and, because of a surgical complication, he had to occlude the anterior choroidal artery on one side. To his surprise, he noted that the patient's tremor improved on the other side. This work led to the development of surgical treatments and, more recently, deep brain stimulation for Parkinson's disease.[1]

In 1982, neurologist William Langston saw six young patients with acute onset of Parkinson's disease following intake of synthetic heroin.[2] Acute onset of the disease had never been previously described. It was discovered that all six had been exposed to a batch of heroin which contained the neurotoxin MPTP (1-methyl-4-phenyl-1,2,3,6-tetrahydropyridine), which is specifically toxic to the nerve cells that are defective in Parkinson's disease. The discovery was important for developing animal models of the disease and enhancing our understanding of its origins.[3] The story of Langston's work is well narrated in his book, *The Case of the Frozen Addicts*.[4]

Morris Bender, a teacher of mine at the Mount Sinai School of Medicine, had a very busy clinical practice in Manhattan. In the 1970s, it was not uncommon for him to have more than 50 patients in the hospital at one time. This was only possible because of the work of the residents who supported him. He had been interested in cortical aspects of sensory function for many years. He collected data from patients in his office and published a report at the age of 77 in the *Journal of Neurological Sciences*.[4] He did not need a laboratory or a gaggle of mice to complete the work.

Neurologists, neurosurgeons, and neuroradiologists frequently perform interventional procedures in the care of acute stroke victims.[5] As discussed in Lesson 39, it is not enough to conclude that a stroke was caused by a thrombosis. Perhaps the factor responsible for the event can be deduced from research on the thrombus itself. This scenario is an example of how a clinician without a laboratory could be involved in research. It may very well be that a researcher studying stroke in mice or cats has never thought of the possibility of performing molecular assessment of stroke in humans.

Many other examples of the importance of clinical descriptions of disease could be mentioned. James Parkinson's book is another example of an important contribution made primarily through observation (Lesson 50).[6,7]

James Parkinson (1755–1824): A Person to Know

Parkinson was an English surgeon, geologist, and politician[6] He followed his father into a medical practice in London. His interests included paleontology, and several species of fossil organisms are named after him. Revolutionary politics was also an area of his interest. He provided early descriptions of gout and perforation of the appendix. In 1817, he published a short book, *An Essay on the Shaking Palsy*, which reported his observations of three of his own patients and three persons that he had seen on the street. He described the characteristic tremor and postural difficulties in the disease named after him. The book is a classic example of a comprehensive disease description (a PDF is freely available).[7]

References

1. Das K, Benzil DL, Rovit RL, Murali R, Couldwell WT. Irving S. Cooper (1922–1985): A pioneer in functional neurosurgery. *J Neurosurg*. 1998 Nov;89(5):865–73. doi:10.3171/jns.1998.89.5.0865. PMID: 9817430.
2. Langston JW. The MPTP story. *J Parkinsons Dis*. 2017;7(s1):S11–S19. doi:10.3233/JPD-179006
3. Langston JW, Palfreman J. *The Case of the Frozen Addicts* (2nd ed.). Pantheon Books; 2014.
4. Bender MB, Stacy C, Cohen J. Agraphesthesia: A disorder of directional cutaneous kinesthesia or a disorientation in cutaneous space. *J Neurol Sci*. 1982 Mar;53(3):531–55. doi:10.1016/0022-510x(82)90249-0. PMID: 6279783.
5. Tonomura S, Ihara M, Friedland RP. Microbiota in cerebrovascular disease: A key player and future therapeutic target. *J Cereb Blood Flow Metab*. 2020 Jul;40(7):1368–80. doi:10.1177/0271678X20918031. Epub 2020 Apr 20. PMID: 32312168; PMCID: PMC7308516.
6. Lewis C. *The Enlightened Mr. Parkinson*. Pegasus; 2017.
7. Parkinson J. An essay on the shaking palsy. Neuropsychiatry Classics. *J Neuropsychiatry Clin Neurosci*. 2002;14:2. https://psychiatryonline.org/doi/pdf/10.1176/jnp.14.2.223

SECTION VII
ETHICS

Lesson 94
Never Whisper in the Presence of Wrong

> Never whisper in the presence of wrong.
> —Bernard Lown[1]

As physicians our responsibility is not limited only to our patients but to society as a whole. Social factors account for 80% of health outcomes.[2] Poor availability of healthcare, poverty, systemic racism, and limited educational and occupational opportunities all have enormous impact on health. We must look beyond the individual patient and see what social factors are involved in health and disease and what can be done about them.

Physicians for Social Responsibility (PSR) is a US organization led by physicians serving to protect the public from nuclear proliferation, climate change, and environmental hazards. It was founded Boston, in 1961, by Bernard Lown, Victor Sidel, and H. Jack Geiger and others. The organization has publicized the hazards of nuclear war and environmental pollution. The work of PSR facilitated the founding of the International Physicians for the Prevention of Nuclear War (IPPNW) in 1980. PSR shared in the 1985 Nobel Peace Prize awarded to the IPPNW for "spreading authoritative information and by creating an awareness of the catastrophic consequences of atomic warfare." PSR continues to work for the elimination of nuclear weapons as well as gun control.

The importance of the social aspects of healthcare are simplified by the inspiring stories of Victor Sidel, H. Jack Geiger, and Bernard Lown.

Victor Sidel (1931–2018): A Person to Know[3]

Sidel was an American physician and President of the American Public Health Association (APHA). He was active in raising awareness of the danger of nuclear proliferation as a public health issue. He was arrested along with 138 other people at a protest organized by the APHA at a nuclear test site in Nevada in 1986. As Chairman of the Department of Social Medicine at Montefiore Medical Center in New York, he trained students and community members about the social factors that influence health. He viewed health as a basic human right. Following Sidel's passing, his associate Barry Levy said, "I can still hear him saying there cannot be health without peace and social justice and there cannot be peace and social justice without health."³

H. Jack Geiger (1925–2020): A Person to Know⁴

Geiger was a physician who believed that physicians had a responsibility to work to improve social problems. He was a lifelong advocate for human rights and helped to start two anti-war physician groups that shared in Nobel Peace Prizes. In addition, he was a cofounder of the concept of "social medicine," the idea that doctors should use their expertise and moral authority not just to treat illness but also to change the conditions that made people sick in the first place: poverty, hunger, discrimination, joblessness, and lack of education.³

Bernard Lown (1921–2021): A Person to Know

Lown was an American cardiologist, humanitarian, and developer of the defibrillator for cardiac resuscitation and the cardioverter for repairing arrhythmias (disordered heart rhythms). He won the 1985 Nobel Peace Prize on behalf of the IPPNW, an organization he co-founded. He was also active in arranging for the rehabilitation of injured children following the war in Vietnam. His work established the importance of getting hospitalized heart disease patients out of bed as soon as possible.⁵

Drs. Sidel, Geiger, and Lown coauthored an important paper in the *New England Journal of Medicine* in 1962 which summarized the devastating effects of a thermonuclear attack on the state of Massachusetts, showing that comparisons to past disasters are inappropriate. In their proposed scenario, they projected that there would be 1,000 injured persons for every surviving physician.⁶

> I want to prevent the wounds, not simply treat them.³
>
> —Victor Seidel

> [P]oor health care and poor health so profoundly limit opportunities ... for the full realization of one's potential ... justice in health care is good for the public's health, and the public's good health, in turn, broadens opportunities and facilitates a more just society.
>
> —H. Jack Geiger⁴

> We go into medicine to make a difference, and we are in a unique position to do so. You cannot be committed to health without being engaged in social struggle for health.⁷
>
> —Bernard Lown

References

1. Lown B. *Never whisper in the presence of wrong*. International Physicians or the Prevention of Nuclear War, Cambridge; 1993.
2. Deng I, Shih P. Social determinants of health the unaddressed variable accounting for 80% of health outcomes. Care Journey blog. https://carejourney.com/social-determinants-of-health/. Accessed Nov 3, 2023.
3. Sanomir R. Dr. Victor Sidel, public health champion, is dead at 86. *New York Times*, Feb 7, 2018.
4. Obituary. H. Jack Geiger, doctor who fought social ills, dies at 95. *New York Times*, Dec 28, 2020.
5. YouTube. Bernard Lown video, Keynote Lecture, Lown Institute. https://www.youtube.com/watch?v=zU6hyxBcY3s&t=740s. Accessed August 2024.
6. Sidel VW, Geiger HJ, Lown B. The medical consequences of thermonuclear war. II. The physician's role in the post-attack period. *N Engl J Med*. 1962 May 31;266:1137–45. doi:10.1056/NEJM196205312662205. PMID: 13912536.
6. Levy BS, Sidel VW. *Social Injustice and Public Health*, 2nd ed. Oxford University Press; 2013.
7. Lown B. *The Lost Art of Healing*. Ballantine Books; 1999.

Lesson 95
You Are Responsible for Your Actions; You Cannot Let Others Take Responsibility for You

Julius Hallervorden (1882–1965) was a German neuropsychiatrist who, with Hugo Spatz, described a rare inherited disorder in 1922 that featured brain iron accumulation. It was called Hallervorden-Spatz disease. In the 1930, he joined the Nazi Party and, in 1938, he became the head of the Neuropathology Department of the Kaiser Wilhelm Institute for Brain Research. He actively participated in a genocidal program code-named T4 involving the murder of hundreds of mentally and physically disabled German children and adults.[1,2] After the war Hallervorden said the following concerning his participation in the T4 program, "Look here now, boys. If you are going to kill all those people, at least take the brains out so that the material can be utilized. They asked me, 'How many can you examine?' and so I told them... 'the more the better.'" He also said, "Where they came from and how they came to me was really none of my business." We are at all times the ones responsible for our own actions. We cannot allow the misguided policies of others to excuse our activities. There is a powerful movie based on Hallervorden's crimes called *Aktion T4*.

Hugo Spatz was also guilty of collaboration with Nazi atrocities.[2] Because of the crimes of Hallervorden and Spatz, the disease they named is now known as now *pantothenate kinase-associated neurodegeneration*.

The editors of *Lancet* formed a commission in 2021 to enhance awareness of the crimes of Nazi doctors during the Holocaust.[3] They noted that more than 200,000 people were murdered because of perceived mental impairments. Also, more than half of Germany's non-Jewish doctors were members of the Nazi Party. Their crimes cannot be forgiven because they were carrying out government policies, of course.

Any personal example of mine concerning the pressure of conforming to the activities of a group will appear trivial in comparison to the story of Hallervorden and Spatz. I present this story below just as an example of the need for independent thinking. I served on an National Institute of Health (NIH) committee reviewing grants for postdoctoral fellowships. One application proposed to inject local anesthesia into a radial nerve in the wrist of volunteers to induce temporary loss of sensation in one hand while functional MRI (fMRI) was done to study the plasticity of the activity in the contralateral sensory cortex. The grant did not discuss the safety of the procedure. The primary reviewers of the grant were two PhD neuroscientists.

There were 20 reviewers in the room, and I was the only one who had an MD degree. Although I was not an assigned reviewer of the grant, I pointed out to the group that injection of local anesthesia into a peripheral nerve was not entirely without risk. When such a procedure is necessary for clinical indications, it is certainly appropriate. However, in the case of this application, it was being done in healthy persons who had no medical indication for having the nerve block. I pointed out that nerves can be injured following regional anesthetic techniques, although such complications were not common.

I raised these concerns and stated that I could not vote to approve the grant since the investigators had not discussed the issue of safety in the application. I was told by the chair of the committee that the safety issues were previously considered by the Institutional Review Board at the home institution of the principal investigator and that the current review committee (of which I was a part) was not responsible for review of the ethical issues concerning the procedure. I said that I could not give up my responsibility to consider the ethics of the research. I affirmed my vote to not fund the project. Everyone else in the room gave the project high scores.

Recently I was asked if I would like to serve as a ringside physician during a boxing match. I would be well paid for a few hours sitting by the boxing ring assessing the health of their combatants. I declined, of course, because the goal of boxing is damage to the nervous system (that's called a "knockout"). In June 2001, in New York City, the boxer Beethaeven Scottland died of head injuries received during a fight. During the fight, Cornell University neurologist Barry Jordan was at ringside.[4] Dr. Jordan was the Chief Medical Officer of the New York State Athletic Commission.

In November 2013, Russian boxer Magomed Abdusalamov lost a fight at the New York Madison Square Garden and was cleared of brain injury by Dr. Jordan after the fight was concluded. It was later found that the boxer had an intracranial hematoma (blood clot). He received intensive care and survived with significant neurological disability.

I believe that the presence of a neurologist at the ringside is unethical because it implies that the physician is able to somehow monitor the safety of the participants. Head injuries are bad for the brain. Aside from the acute consequences of boxing disasters, as shown in these two cases, it is well known that head injuries are a risk factor for chronic traumatic encephalopathy (CTE).[5] This condition is associated with all forms of head injury including boxing and American football, and it can cause progressive untreatable dementia, depression, suicide, agitation, and loss of motor control.

You cannot attribute responsibility for your actions to others. If something is wrong, it is wrong regardless of whether some committee or powerful individual has said it is the right thing to do. **Do not be coerced into group think. The importance of including the Holocaust in medical education is reviewed in a paper in Science in 2023.**[3]

Unanimity of opinion may be fitting for a church, for the frightened or greedy victims of some (ancient, or modern) myth, or for the weak and willing followers of some tyrant. Variety of opinion is necessary for objective knowledge. And a method that encourages variety is also the only method that is comparable with a humanitarian outlook.

—Paul Feyerabend[6]

No injury to the head is too trifling to be despised.
—Attributed to Hippocrates (460–370 BC), Greek physician

References

1. Friedland RP. Julius Hallervorden. *Neurology.* 1993 Jul;43(7):1453. doi:10.1212/wnl.43.7.1453. PMID: 832716
2. Voges L, Kupsch A. Renaming of Hallervorden-Spatz disease: The second man behind the name of the disease. *J Neural Transm (Vienna).* 2021 Nov;128(11):1635–40. doi:10.1007/s00702-021-02408-x. Epub 2021 Oct 16. PMID: 34655340; PMCID: PMC8536572.
3. Vogel G. Medical education must include the field's Nazi past, expert panel urges. *Science.* 2023 Nov. 10.10.1126/science.adm8848
4. Wong E. Medical examiner is still trying to determine exact cause of boxer's death. *New York Times.* Jul 5, 2001.
5. McKee AC, Abdolmohammadi B, Stein TD. The neuropathology of chronic traumatic encephalopathy. *Handb Clin Neurol.* 2018;158:297–307. doi:10.1016/B978-0-444-63954-7.00020-0. PMID. 30482357.
6. Feyerabend P. *Against Method*, Verso, 4th Edition. 2010.

Lesson 96
The Need To Believe in the Guilty Victim

It is deeply established in human behavior to believe that people who suffer deserve their suffering. This is part of the Buddhist and Hindu concept of karma (your actions determine what happens to you). The idea of karma specifies that you will be rewarded for good actions, and you will suffer for evil actions—what happens to a person happens because they caused it with their actions. This principle is also a part of Judeo-Christian beliefs: suffering may be God's punishment for past sins. The idea that parental sins or transgressions influence the life of the children is deeply embedded in Greek mythology. Homer explained that the consequences of paternal indiscretions seriously affect the life of the children (Iliad, AD 170). In Greece, Rome, and elsewhere, disease was believed to be a result of a personal fault or an ancestral crime resulting in guilt. It was taught throughout the Middle Ages (and widely believed) that the poor were poor and the king was the king because it was God's will.

These views have not been completely eliminated with modernity. The American psychiatrist Karl Menninger has said, "Illness is in part what the world has done to a victim, but in a large part it is what the victim has done with his world and with himself." As outlined by the American novelist Susan Sontag in her essay *Illness as Metaphor*,[1] this view inappropriately puts the blame on the patient and impairs her ability to seek proper treatment. An extreme view is presented in Samuel Butler's 1872 novel, *Erewhon*, in which disease is punished as a crime.

A 1998 psychological research study investigated these matters. Research volunteers watched videos showing people being questioned and punished with electric shocks for wrong answers.[2] The victims who received the shocks were actually actors pretending to be in pain. Volunteers preferred to interact with those who were not shocked compared to the ones who were shocked. These results contributed to the concept that there is a need to believe in the guilty victim.

In medicine, there is a tendency for healthcare workers to blame patients when the patient appears to have contributed to the problem.[3,4] For example, an obese person may be blamed for excessive eating and an alcoholic for irresponsible drinking. This lack of compassion is unfortunate, erroneous, and dangerous. Recent studies show that obese persons may have different gut bacteria than others, which causes them to be better at harvesting nutrition from their food. Similar evidence indicates that both alcoholism and smoking have genetic influences.

Many years ago, I participated in a survey of farmers in rural Arkansas analyzing the effects of toxic exposures. I was disturbed that many of the people I examined did not wash before coming to the appointment and had dirty and foul-smelling clothes. A colleague told me what should have been obvious—that they were poor and may not have other clothes or access to hot water. This is an example of improperly blaming the patient.

The false belief that some of our patients deserve their suffering or are personally responsible is a dangerous defense mechanism which allows us to remain separate and protects us from the frightening realization that the patient's disease could happen to us. The truth is that we must understand that we are just like our patients—we are products of our genes and environment, as our patients are, and we need to treat them with this understanding.[3,4]

It is not helpful to be angry at unvaccinated people in the era of COVID-19, even though their irresponsible decision to not be vaccinated may be responsible for their deaths. A *New England Journal of Medicine* editorial considered a man dying of COVID who had chosen to be unvaccinated from the perspective of his ICU physician. "Labeling him as one of 'the unvaccinated' and bringing my anger into the room served only to distract me, preventing me from finding the compassion and connection that allow me to feel whole as I return each day to an environment rife with suffering."[5]

An important aspect of the need to believe in the guilty victim is the fear and pain caused by the reality of illness. The practice of medicine involves contact with the sick, which is a reminder of our own mortality. It is a defense mechanism to diminish the fearful implications of the illness of another by believing that it could not happen to us. It is necessary to accept the reality that it can and will happen to us, because the practice of medicine does not come with any guarantees of our own personal health and well-being.[6] This has been expressed by a phrase I heard years ago from the disability community of Berkeley, California. They refer to healthy nondisabled persons as "TABs": Temporarily Able-Bodied.

We cannot allow our compassion for the patient to be limited because of the false belief that the patient is responsible for the disease.

References

1. Sontag S. *Illness as Metaphor*. Doubleday; 1972: 46.
2. Lerner MJ, Montada L. An overview. In Montada L., Lerner MJ (eds.), *Responses to Victimizations and Belief in a Just World*. Critical Issues in Social Justice. Springer; 1998: 247–269. https://doi.org/10.1007/978-1-4757-6418-5_1
3. Wu A. How to stop yourself from blaming the patient. OP-MED; 2021 Mar 4. https://opmed.doximity.com/articles/how-to-stop-yourself-from-blaming-the-patient. Accessed Oct 31, 2023.
4. Roberts K. *The Psychology of Victim-Blaming*. Atlantic; 2016.
5. Garfinkel AC. From resentment to reconnection: Reflections on caring for the unvaccinated. *N Engl J Med*. 2022 Apr 14;386(15):1394–5. doi:10.1056/NEJMp2119720. Epub 2022 Apr 9. PMID: 35417934.
6. Grady D. "I had never faced the reality of death": A surgeon becomes a patient. *New York Times*, Jun 3, 2021. https://www.nytimes.com/2021/06/03/health/covid-19-diagnosis-surgeon.html. Accessed Aug 2024.

Lesson 97
Compassion Is Part of Our Fundamental Nature

Just as evolution has enhanced our appreciation of stories (Lesson 3), natural selection has also supported our capacity for compassion. *Compassion* is defined as the feeling of sorrow or deep tenderness for one who is suffering or experiencing misfortune and of suffering with another. "The feeling or emotion, when a person is moved by the suffering or distress of another, and by the desire to relieve it" (*Oxford English Dictionary*). The feeling of compassion is similar to sympathy.

If we imagine human societies in the past 100,000 years, it is obvious that the capacity to be kind to others and to understand and appreciate their feelings is beneficial for human survival. If person A is kind to the children of person B, it is likely that person B will be more kind to the children of person A. In this way, it is clear that **compassion is part of our fundamental nature.** The practice of compassion is not so much a matter of learning but rather a process of appreciating that it is already present within us.

Compassion must begin with compassion for ourselves. As expressed by His Holiness the Dalai Lama, "Joy is compassion turned inward." Once we have been able to manifest kindness to and understanding of our own suffering then we can better express compassion to others.

Notably, compassion can be hindered by several mechanisms. For example, intellectualization provides thoughts and concepts which prevent us from feeling (see Lesson 9). Rationalization can provide us with reasons why persons are suffering, and these reasons can block our experience of compassion (as noted in Lesson 96).

Compassion can also be inhibited by fear, which can be experienced in many ways, "If I allow myself to sympathize with this person too much I will have trouble controlling my emotions." Although being compassionate does not mean that we sob on the patient's shoulder, we should allow ourselves to be aware of our own human responses to the suffering of others. Harvard physician Jerome Groopman has said "to become immune to feeling … is to diminish the full role of the physician as a healer and relegate him to a single dimension of his job, that of a tactician. If we feel our emotions deeply, we risk recoiling or breaking down. If we erase our emotions, however, we fail to care *for* the patient. We face a paradox: feeling prevents us from being blind to our patient's soul but risks blinding us to what is wrong with him."[1] We need to be balanced and learn how to express our compassion without losing our ability to provide care.

Our ability to express compassion can also be limited by the fear that the patient encounter will take too much time. The importance of listening and being there for the patient must be recognized at all levels of the healthcare system. In the United States, the system is currently focused on enhancing billing and not enriching opportunities for patient–doctor communication.

It may also be feared that being compassionate will make one appear unprofessional. Compassion can be compromised by many of the forms of bias (Lessons 51–53). We all need to recognize our potential for bias, learn to accept and recognize our capacity for compassion, and express our sympathy through our actions.

Our compassion may also be limited at times because of the immense volume of suffering. The February 2023 Turkey-Syria earthquake killed 59,259 people and was the deadliest natural disaster in modern history. Common response to such a catastrophe is resignation and the thought that there is nothing that could possibly be done to help (psychic numbing). It needs to be understood that what is required of us is to do what we can—we are not responsible for fixing every problem all by ourselves. University of Oregon psychologist Paul Slovic refers to this problem as "pseudoinefficiency" because there is something people can do.[2] A similar inappropriate restriction of compassion may be observed in physicians caring for patients who have intractable illnesses and disabilities.

A teaching from Judaism guides us. "Do not be daunted by the enormity of the world's grief. Do justly, now. Love mercy, now. Walk humbly, now. You are not obligated to complete the work, but neither are you free to abandon it."[3]

There can also be times when compassion is inhibited because the physician does not know what to say. When confronted with progressive which can no longer be alleviated there may be a tendency to avoid contact. It is vital to understand that our presence is a significant factor. **Compassion can be expressed by the critical act of listening and being there** (Lesson 72).

The capacity for compassion should have no limits. All our patients are suitable recipients of our compassion. The practice of meditation is a valuable opportunity for enhancing our compassion.[4]

> Beware of the differences that blind us to the unity that binds us.[5]
> —Huston Smith, religious scholar

References

1. Groopman J. *How Doctors Think*. Mariner Books; 2008: 17.
2. Resnick B. A psychologist explains the limits of human compassion, *Vox* 2017;9:5.
3. Pirkei Avot. Commentary on Micah 6:8 by Rabbi Trifon. https://reformjudaism.org/beliefs-practices/spirituality/3-jewish-reminders-when-world-seems-overwhelming. Accessed Aug 2024.
4. Hanh Thich Nat. *You Are Here: Discovering the Magic of the Present Moment*. Shambala Press; 2001.
5. Smith H. *Why Religion Matters*. Harper; 2006.

Lesson 98
The Myth of Progress

The myth of progress is the idea that improvements in the human condition are happening and will continue. English physician Montague Eder wrote in 1932 that "the myth of progress states that civilization has moved, is moving, and will move in a desirable direction. Progress is inevitable."[1] This idea that all progress is improvement is a variety of the bias in favor of new ideas.

The myth of progress has been criticized because technological advancements can have negative effects. Realizing that the concept of progress is a myth can help us to appreciate the complex outcomes caused by medical and scientific changes that occur with time.

Consider these scenarios:

- New diagnostic techniques can negatively impact a patient's life. Some persons informed of a high Alzheimer's disease risk may actually never have the disease affect them in their lifetime (Lesson 17).
- New drugs can have untoward effects which are not apparent from clinical trials (such as rofecoxib, a promising COX-2-selective nonsteroidal anti-inflammatory drug that was found to increase the risk of heart attacks and stroke. At one time more than 80 million persons worldwide were taking the drug.)
- New technologies such as the electronic health record can provide such a massive amount of information (information toxicity) that pivotal features of our patient's problems may be missed (Lesson 19).
- Online publication has vastly expanded the number of medical and scientific journals available. This has seriously diluted the scientific literature, making it harder to follow progress in science. Many new journals have poor academic standards.[2]
- The availability of data-sharing involving global consortia can create vast amounts of data that require expert statistical analysis because of the danger of confounding and erroneous conclusions due to multiple comparisons. Similar problems exist in research studies in which large amounts of data are acquired with small subject sizes.
- I know more about molecular biology than my teachers did because I have been witness to the scientific progress of the past several decades, which they did not experience. However, their experience was different from mine, and, in many ways, it was deeper than mine. For example, before advances of imaging in the

1980s, the physical exam was the key to diagnosis. Currently the physical exam is not properly appreciated as an important contributor to patient understanding.
- The morbidity and mortality (sickness and death) of infectious diseases in low- and middle-income countries has declined significantly in the past 50 years. However, lifestyle changes involving diet, social support, and physical exercise are having negative effects on health in many areas. The risk of obesity, hypertension, and coronary heart disease is growing in Africa. It is estimated that cardiovascular disease will become the leading cause of death in Africa, overtaking infectious diseases by 2030.

Of course, progress in medicine and science cannot be canceled, and we would not want to do so if we could. Great improvements are being made in understanding disease and scientific problems. What is important is to keep in mind is that progress is not 100% beneficial, and the idea that progress is uniformly beneficial is a myth. We need to pay attention to the key elements of awareness of the patient's needs. And we need to pay attention to how we think about scientific problems so that we put healthcare into the context of our patient's lives.

References

1. David Eder, Montague. General: M. D. Eder. "The Myth of Progress." *The British Journal of Medical Psychology*, 1932, Vol. XII, p. 1. *International Journal of Psychoanalysis* 1932;14:399
2. Singh Chawla D. The undercover academic keeping tabs on "predatory" publishing. *Nature*. 2018 Mar 22;555(7697):422–3. doi:10.1038/d41586-018-02921-2. PMID: 29565386.

Lesson 99
Don't Be Ageist

Ageism is a form of discrimination against persons of a certain age, usually older people.[1] Long-standing cultural beliefs include negative and inaccurate stereotypes about older persons. Although old persons are honored in Christian, Muslim, Jewish, Buddhist, and Hindu traditions, there are often ways in which the "honoring" process is misguided. Older persons may be respected, housed, and fed without attention to their social and psychological needs. That is, they may be honored with deference (respect), but without influence, the ability to guide their own lives.

It was widely assumed until the 1970s that severe memory loss in later life was caused by hardening of the arteries in the neck, without experimental evidence. The condition was referred to as "senility," a worthless term which means "old." Older persons who had what we now call Alzheimer's disease were largely ignored because it was believed that everyone developed dementia when they got to be old. We now know this to be mistaken.

Life expectancy is increasing in many areas of the world, and many countries have low birth rates, meaning that the average age of the population is rising. This is especially the case in Japan and the Republic of Korea. The rise in the number of older persons in worldwide populations has not been accompanied by increased resources for the special needs of older persons. The field of geriatrics, which is relatively recent, is suffering a shortage of workers because of the lack of government support in the United States. The US Department of Health predicts a shortage of almost 27,000 geriatricians by 2025.[2] Responses to the aging of global populations have been inadequate around the globe.

An important component of ageism is discrimination against women because most old people are female. (According to the United Nations, in 2019, 61% of people 80 years of age or older were female.)

An important perspective on aging is presented in the paper, "Can we afford medical care for Alice C."[3] An 88-year-old woman who had relatively rapid onset of difficulty breathing was given emergency treatment, including resuscitation, even though she was initially thought to be "as good as dead." One medical resident asked "is it appropriate to give such expensive treatment to an 88-year-old woman who is probably going to die anyway?" This question implies that age-related criteria need to be applied to the availability of medical care. Alice C. was found to have pneumonia and was treated with antibiotics during a 10-day ICU stay. She later went home and was able to resume her normal activities for at least another 5 years.

Two other cases of older patients who did well despite complex comorbidities are described in the paper "An act of futility, or Pascal's wager?"[4]

In 1984, the governor of Colorado, Richard Lamm, said "We've got a duty to die and get out of the way with all of our machines and artificial hearts and everything else like that and let the other society, our kids, build a reasonable life."[5] This outrageously biased position fails to realize that healthcare is a right of old as well as young persons. It is only a short cognitive moment to go from denial of care to the elderly to eugenics and other crimes against humanity.*

The 97-year-old father of a friend of mine drove his car to the shop to be repaired, walked across the street to the bus, and was hit by a car that had gone through a stop sign. He suffered a closed head injury, cerebral contusions, and an intracranial hematoma. His prognosis was poor because of his age and bleeding in the brain. He received intensive care and rehabilitation and was discharged to his home, where he received personal assistance and enjoyed contact with his family. He died at the age of 108. It is important to understand that our ability to predict outcomes is flawed, and everyone deserves an opportunity to exceed age-based expectations.

What makes life worth living varies from person to person at different stages of the life course. Younger people may have trouble understanding that an older person who has limited mobility, vision, and hearing may still have a life filled with joy and meaning. There is a pervasive tendency for many people to fail to appreciate the preciousness of life at every age. There are, of course, occasions of severe illness and disability when decisions about the appropriateness of care must be made. These decisions should not be made based on age alone.

Age discrimination is also seen throughout the world in regard to retirement decisions. Medical school faculty are forced to retire at 65–67 in many places in Europe and Japan. Several of the investigators I know who were forced to abandon their laboratory and funding retained their productivity into their later years of life. My own father-in-law was a school principal in India and was forced to retire at the age of 55. At his retirement celebration he was honored with the gift of a cane even though he had no use for it whatsoever.

My view is that university faculty who are not productive should be made to retire without regard to their age. Older faculty who are productive should be treasured for their contributions.

In 2014, 57-year-old oncologist and bioethicist Ezekiel Emanuel asserted that he hoped to die at 75 years of age.[6] He argued that society and families will be better off "if nature takes its course swiftly and promptly." He has a distorted and erroneous view of aging. Many persons retain good physical and mental function until their 80s and 90s. Nobel laureate Eric Kandel authored a book at the age of 89. Emanuel forgets the pivotal fact that although cognitive and physical functions decline with age, variability increases. That means that there are persons over 60, over 70, and over

---

* *Eugenics* is the method of controlling reproduction of humans to increase the occurrence of inherited features thought to be desirable and decrease the occurrence of undesirable features.

80 who are functioning just as well as many persons who are 20–30 years younger. He also ignores the truth that many aged persons have further contributions to make to the world.

I do not accept the proposition that because healthcare resources are limited, they should not be extended to persons who have already had an opportunity to live a full life. What could be more important than caring for a 82-year-old with pneumonia who may have more than 10 years of life left if adequately treated? Would it be better for government expenses to be used for fireworks at July 4th celebrations? Or the landscaping of highways? All persons are of value, at all ages. Older people are no of less value than younger persons because of their physical and cognitive changes.

My most fundamental belief is that life is precious. This belief applies to persons of all ages.

References

1. Butler RN. Combating ageism. *Int Psychogeriatr.* 2009 Apr;21(2):211. doi:10.1017/S104161020800731X. Epub 2008 Sep 26. PMID: 18817584.
2. American Association of Medical Colleges. Prescription for America's elder boom: Every doctor learns geriatric. https://www.aamc.org/news/prescription-america-s-elder-boom-every-doctor-learns-geriatrics. Accessed Oct 21, 2023.
3. Levinsky NG. Can we afford medical care for Alice C? *Lancet.* 1998 Dec 5;352(9143):1849–51. doi:10.1016/S0140-6736(98)07555-2. PMID: 9851402.
4. Hutchins AM, Windham DM. An act of futility or Pascal's wager? *Clin Pathol Res J.* 2020;4:1.
5. Governor Lamb asserts elderly, if every ill, have "duty to die." *New York Times.* Mar 29, 1984. https://www.nytimes.com/1984/03/29/us/gov-lamm-asserts-elderly-if-very-ill-have-duty-to-die.html. Accessed Aug 2024.
6. Emanuel E. Why I hope to die at 75. *The Atlantic.* 2014.

Epilogue

The key factor in critical thinking is asking questions and paying attention to the question. Is it the right question? Is it properly framed? Does it contain errors or biases? Is it important? Is it trivial? Does it already have an answer? Is it a good question for me to consider? Is it a good question for someone else but not me?

The timing of questioning is also vital. The best strategy is to start right away asking questions and never stop. Questioning is the key to critical thinking and also the key to good patient care. Questions should focus on the patient and not on our own thoughts or on the medical record. All of our patients' stories are different, and we need to make sure that our responses account for the patient's uniqueness.

We must be properly attentive if we are to learn what the patient has to teach. The decisions we make about what is going on and what we are to do must be based on what we have learned through our attention and questioning. The decision should not be based only on our knowledge or our preconceived ideas, biases, and false expectations. **We can best learn what the patient has to tell us and we can best express our humanity by asking the right questions.** Questioning is the basic component of critical thinking.

Have you heard about the two monks from different monasteries who were old friends who shared a great fondness for cigars. Once each year when they had a chance to visit, they would pray together and light up. Eventually, however, they became concerned that their habit might be sinful, and they each resolved to ask their respective superiors for guidance. When they met again, one was puffing away. "But the head of my monastery told me it was not allowed to smoke during my evening prayers," said the other, "What did you ask him?" said the first. "I asked him if it was all right to smoke during my evening prayers, and he said, 'No.'" "Well," said his friend as he blew a perfect smoke ring into the air, "I asked my superior if it was all right to pray during my evening smoke, and he said it was just fine!"[1] The way a question is phrased is essential.

Consider neuromyelitis optica (NMO), a human brain disease affecting the white matter tracts in the brain, spinal cord, and eyes. It is associated with antibodies to the water channel protein aquaporin 4, which cause damage to the white matter. When asked what is the cause of the disease, many physicians say, "antibodies against aquaporin 4." Antibodies to aquaporin 4 are auto-antibodies because they are targeting a host protein. The occurrence of auto-antibodies could happen by a random unfortunate immunological mistake. But many things thought to be random are not random. Consider another possibility: if a protein similar to aquaporin 4 was present in the world, certain people could be exposed and then develop antibodies targeting aquaporin 4. We did a computerized search using a Basic Local Alignment Search Tool (BLAST) of the National Library of Medicine which compared all known protein sequences with the structure of aquaporin 4. We located a protein found in plants which has significant similarity to a region of neuronal aquaporin 4.[2]

To our surprise (drum roll please), the plant protein which has a similarity to neuronal aquaporin 4 is called "aquaporin." It turns out that the structure of these water channel proteins is evolutionarily conserved between kingdoms (between plants and animals). Of course, this should not be surprising considering the importance of water balance for both plants and animals. It has been suggested that patients with NMO should avoid plant aquaporins present in spinach, corn, soybeans, and tomatoes. (We have also found significant examples of surprising similarity of protein structure involving plant viruses and brain proteins.[3])

I have asserted that the formation of questions should consider evolution. Does this refer only to structural features? What about emotions? Posttraumatic stress disorder (PTSD) is a condition that follows an experience involving witnessing a frightening, terrifying, or dangerous event. Why is the power and persistence of depression and anxiety related to PTSD so remarkable? Imagine an early ancestor of yours, perhaps 15,000 years ago, who was exploring a new territory and found a lovely waterfall with a profusion of lilies. She goes back to her group and tells her family about the flowers. And the next day she goes to back to pick some lilies and is attacked by a bear who is about to kill her when a crocodile frightens off the bear, allowing her to escape. The memory of the first scenario (the lilies) is not critical to her survival. On the other hand, remembering where the bear attack took place could save her life. Evolution has developed mechanisms whereby memories formed during stressful events are more powerfully represented in the brain than are memories of trivial events. It is adaptive for such memories to be especially salient. The neural mechanisms of memory involve neural connections, and memories of stressful events involve more synapses, neurotransmitter receptors, and representation in neural networks than do events which are not life-threatening.[4] This evolutionary viewpoint suggests that PTSD is not only a psychological reaction to stress. It also represents a powerful change in brain structure. The greater strength of memories of stressful events is adaptive and favored by evolution. When we question the durability of PTSD, we should consider human evolution as well as individual psychology.

I have had a personal experience which illustrates the role of stress in memory. As a 10-year-old, I was allowed to walk two blocks by myself to get a haircut. I would pay the barber 25 cents and then walk home. One day I forgot to bring money and, when I told the barber I could not pay him, he yelled at me. Every time I go to have my hair cut, I feel a small twinge of anxiety and check if I have money to pay the barber. Of course, the stress involved in this event was trivial, but it was enough to change my lifelong response to barbers.

We are often afraid to ask questions and interrogate problems deeply. Not infrequently, students are taught earlier in their education to be quiet, not make trouble, and not ask questions. Many of us learn in school that we must not ask questions which challenge the prevailing view or which may reveal the ignorance of the teacher. We all need to reject this fear of questioning.

There is a lovely story about Isidore Rabi, who won the Nobel Prize in Physics in 1944 for the discovery of nuclear magnetic resonance. He credited his mother with his scientific accomplishments. Rabi said that this mother made him a scientist. Other mothers would ask his friends, when they come home from school "What did you learn today?" His mother would ask instead, "Did you ask any good questions today?"

As we have seen many times in this book, critical thinking requires courage and a willingness to be independent. It is important that critical arguments be complemented with creative ideas. Asking questions with ferocity (Lesson 4) can lead to all sorts of difficulties. But this independence is the key to progress in medicine and science.

As a guide to critical thinking, we should remember the wisdom of Sydney Brenner, who suggested a "don't worry" hypothesis (Lesson 80). Don't expect all your ideas to explain everything.

Are some questions improper? What do you think is the value of a hypothesis which cannot be tested? Austrian-British philosopher of science Karl Popper (1902–1994) proposed a *falsification principle*, that a scientific theory must be testable and able to be proved false. By this measure, an untestable hypothesis is not scientific. A key matter is untestable according to whom? I may have an idea and not know how to test it. And I may meet with others who also cannot see how to test it. But there may be someone I do not know who can see how to test the hypothesis. The global scientific community is deep and wide. Publication and dissemination of theories can be valuable, even if the theories appear to be untestable. The progress of science is not predictable.

Our pursuit of critical thinking should be a source of joy for each of us to help other people deal with health and disease. Many people do not have the opportunity to develop a life of meaning and significance. The understanding of our great responsibility as providers and scientists will help us to use critical thinking to focus our attention and properly manage our inquiry. As we interact with patients and pursue scientific studies, we have a chance to utilize all our human skills, not only our ability to move, hear, and see, but also our capacity for understanding, comprehension, storytelling, imagination, memory, critical thinking, and, most of all, compassion. Patient care gives us an opportunity to express our humanity on a daily basis.

Practicing critical thinking can be exciting and magnificently rewarding, in terms of both individual accomplishments and contributions to human welfare. With clean socks we can stand on the shoulders of giants and enjoy a magnificent view of the scientific arena (Lesson 74). We must all exercise our shoulder muscles so that we can support the next generations of doctors and scientists who will be standing on our shoulders as well.

> The one thing that really characterized our conversations is that we never restrained ourselves in anything we said—even if it sounded completely stupid. We understood that just uttering something gets it out into the open and that someone else might pick up from that. There are people who will not say anything until they've got it all worked out. I think such people are missing the most important thrill about research—the social interaction, the companionship that comes from two people's minds playing on each other. And I think that's the most important thing. To say it, even if it's completely stupid!"
>
> —Sydney Brenner[5]

> I consider myself mediocre.... The only thing I know of myself is that I like asking stupid questions. Nine out of 10 questions I made and continue to make were/are stupid or nonsense. Yet one out of 10 proved to be good.[6]
>
> —Ryuzo Yanagimachi

Ryuzo Yanagimachi (1928–2023): A Person to Know

Yanagimachi was a Japanese American scientist who developed methods for cloning mice which advanced the technology of transgenic animals (transgenic animals have had their genome altered through genetic engineering). Methods he developed are widely used today in infertility clinics around the world. Early in his career he had trouble finding an academic position in Japan, and he worked as a postdoctoral fellow in Massachusetts. He had difficulty again finding a position in Japan and worked at the University of Hawaii from 1966 to 2005 until he retired at the age of 77. He won numerous prizes and is quoted as saying "Unlike people, nature never lies."

References

1. Cigarforums.net. Accessed May 23, 2023.
2. Vaishnav RA, Liu R, Chapman J, Roberts AM, Ye H, Rebolledo-Mendez JD, Tabira T, Fitzpatrick AH, Achiron A, Running MP, Friedland RP. Aquaporin 4 molecular mimicry and implications for neuromyelitis optica. *J Neuroimmunol*. 2013 Jul 15;260(1–2):92–8. doi:10.1016/j.jneuroim.2013.04.015. Epub 2013 May 9. PMID: 23664693; PMCID: PMC3682654.
3. Friedland RP. Mechanisms of molecular mimicry involving the microbiota in neurodegeneration. *J Alzheimers Dis*. 2015;45(2):349–62. doi:10.3233/JAD-142841. PMID: 25589730.
4. Toledo F, Carson F. Neurobiological features of posttraumatic stress disorder (PTSD) and their role in understanding adaptive behavior and stress resilience. *Int J Environ Res Public Health*. 2022 Aug 18;19(16):10258. doi:10.3390/ijerph191610258. PMID: 36011896; PMCID: PMC9407950.
5. Pieribone V, Gruber DF. *Aglow in the Dark: The Revolutionary Science of Biofluorescence*. Belknap; 2007.
6. Yanagimachi R. Germ cells and fertilization: Why I studied these topics and what I learned along the path of my study. *Andrology*. 2014 Nov;2(6):787–93. doi:10.1111/j.2047-2927.2014.00238.x. PMID: 25327579.

Quotations on the Nature of the Scientific Endeavor

Ralph Waldo Emerson (1803–1882), American author and philosopher

> Do not go where the path may lead, go instead where there is no path and leave a trail.

Robert Musil (adapted) (1880–1942), Austrian philosopher

> Thirst for knowledge is like an addiction or a yearning for love ... as it throws a character off balance. It is not true that the scientist goes after the truth. It goes there, it goes after him. It is something he suffers from.[1]

Henri Poincare (1854–1912), French mathematician and theoretical physicist

> The subliminal self is in no way inferior to the conscious self; it is not purely automatic; it is capable of discernment; it has tact, delicacy; it knows how to choose, to divine. What do I say? It knows better how to divine than the conscious self, since it succeeds where that has failed.[2]

Martin A. Schwartz, American cell biologist

> We might think of an experiment as a conversation with nature, where we ask a question and listen for an answer, then interpret the answer. This process is personal in that the questions come from us. But by listening for an answer that comes from nature, there is also a way in which it connects to something vastly larger than we are; something that might even be universal.[3]

Albert Szent-Györgyi (1893–1986)

> [I]n spite of all the hard work involved, research is not a systematic occupation but an intuitive artistic vocation.[4]

George Bernard Shaw (1856–1950)

> All great truths begin as blasphemies.[5]

References

1. Musil R. *The Man Without Qualities* (1930–1943). Rowohit Verlag; 1979.
2. Popova M, Popovs M. Tae MArginalian https://www.themarginalian.org/2013/08/15/henri-poincare-on-how-creativity-works/. Accessed Aug 2024.
3. Schwartz MA. The importance of indifference in scientific research. *J Cell Sci.* 2015 Aug 1;128(15):2745–6. doi:10.1242/jcs.174946. Epub 2015 Jul 1. PMID: 26136366; PMCID: PMC6518312.
4. Szent-Györgyi A. Lost in the 20th century. *Ann Rev Biochem.* 1963;32.
5. Shaw GB. *Annajanska, the Bolshevik Empress: A Revolutionary Romancelet* (1917). CreateSpace; 2017.

About the Author

Dr. Friedland is a clinical and research cognitive neurologist devoted to the study of brain disorders associated with aging. He is a graduate of the City College of New York and the Mount Sinai School of Medicine in New York. He worked in the Lawrence Berkeley Laboratory of the University of California, Berkeley, as Chief Neurologist, and was Deputy Clinical Director and Chief of the Section on Brain Aging and Dementia of the National Institute on Aging, NIH. At Case Western Reserve University in Cleveland, he was Professor of Neurology, Psychiatry, and Radiology. In 2008, he joined the faculty of the University of Louisville as Rudd Chair and Professor of Neurology. His work is focused on clinical and biological issues in Alzheimer's disease and related disorders, with collaborators in the United States, the United Kingdom, Israel, and Japan. He has authored or coauthored more than 350 papers, which have been cited over 20,000 times. His book, *Unaging: The Four Factors That Impact Your Aging*, was published by Cambridge University Press in 2022. He lives with his wife, Shivani Nandi, PhD, in Louisville Kentucky.

Index

For the benefit of digital users, indexed terms that span two pages (e.g., 52–53) may, on occasion, appear on only one of those pages.

Figures are indicated by an italic *f* following the page number.

Abdusalamov, Magomed, 253
actions, responsibility for your, 252–53
active reading, 168
Act of Creation, The (Koestler), 207
Adams, Raymond, 13
Adler, Alfred, 163
Adolphus, Gustavus (King), 127
Adrian, Edgar, 233
aducanumab, 116
Advice for a Young Investigator (Ramon y Cajal), 195
affinity bias, 135
Against Method (Feyerabend), 208
ageism, 261–63
    discrimination against older people, 261
    discrimination against women, 261
Aktion T4, 252
alanine aminotransferase (ALT), 35
alcohol abuse, 13
alcohol intake
    patient visit, 29
    pregnancy, 118
Alexander the Great, 110
Alzheimer, Alois, 100, 178, 194–95
Alzheimer's disease, 7, 17, 24–25, 88, 141, 146
    amyloid beta protein PET scan, 49
    apolipoprotein E e4 (Apo E e4), 152–53
    being aware of ignorance, 52
    calcification and, 141
    caring for patient, 182
    communicating diagnosis, 92
    data collection, 225
    dementia, 63
    diagnosis of, 22
    diagnostic service, 116–17
    etiology of, 90
    genes and, 52
    glucose metabolism, 201, 236
    information about genetic risk, 49–50
    motor neuron disease (MND) and, 60–61
    MRI scan, 56
    mutations and early-onset, 115
    neurologist on, 99–100
    new drug for, 110
    nootropics and, 101
    older persons with, 261
    olfactory dysfunction, 241–42
    oral health as risk factor, 66–67
    papers by Fuller and Alzheimer, 179
    pathogenesis, 47
    pathophysiology of, 90
    positron emission tomography (PET), 185
    posterior cortical atrophy variant, 63
    Reagan's diagnosis, 80
    research on, 187
    risk, 259
    risk gene, 90
    role of lifestyle factors, 118
    smoking and, 135
    study of, 214
    telling the truth, 76
    treatment trial, 235–36
amantadine, 25
American Board of Psychiatry and Neurology, 136
American football, head injury, 253
American Heart Journal (journal), 243
American Medical Association, 86
American Neurological Association, 51
American Psychiatric Association, 137–38
American Public Health Association (APHA), 249–50
amyotrophic lateral sclerosis (ALS), 145, 146
anatomy, 58–59
anchoring, 87
anchoring bias, 133, 134
animal models, 114
An Introduction to Experimental Medicine (Bernard), 224
An Introduction to the Study of Experimental Medicine (Bernard), 122
antagonistic pleiotropy, 152–53
antibodies, 137
Antonovsky, Aaron, 66, 67
anxiety, 266
aquaporin, neuronal aquaporin 4 as, 265–66
Archimedes, 207
Aristotle, 110, 142
artificial intelligence (AI), 86, 87–88, 161
    ChatGTP, 87, 183
    generative AI models, 87

Index

ascorbic acid, discovery of, 185
aspartate aminotransferase (AST), 35
astrophysics, 193
atrophy, "stork legs," 62
attention, 159
   medication, 94–95
   mind as powerful tool, 108
attribution errors, 133
availability bias, 132
Avicenna (Ibn Sina), 187–88
   person to know, 188

Babinski sign, 64
Bacon, Sir Francis, 142, 224
   person to know, 142
Banting, Frederick, 233
Basic Local Alignment Search Tool (BLAST), National Library of Medicine, 265
Bellevue Hospital, 37
bell rung, term, 34
Bender, Morris B., 51, 182, 196, 245
benzene, Kekulé on structure, 108
Bernard, Claude, 42, 122, 125, 224, 225
   person to know, 42
Berra, Yogi, 5, 145
Berson, Solomon, 112
Best, Charles, 233
Betadine, 41
Better (Gawande), 14
bias
   affinity bias, 135
   anchoring bias, 133, 134
   availability, 132
   commission bias, 133
   confirmation bias, 132, 134
   desirability, 133
   development of, 131
   diagnosis momentum, 133
   experimenter, 141–42
   favor of common conditions, 136
   favor of new ideas, 132
   favor of rare conditions, 136
   framing bias, 132
   herd mentality, 133
   hindsight bias, 134–35
   implicit bias, 137
   lost actors, 143
   narrative fallacy, 133
   against new ideas, 132
   no clinical experience, 136
   optimism bias, 135
   overconfidence, 132
   sampling bias, 135
   self-serving, 133
   survivorship bias, 143

biochemistry, 223
biology, 173
biomarkers
   Alzheimer's disease, 116–17
   Streptococcus infection, 116
Biophilia (Wilson), 5
bismuth, 30
bismuth poisoning, 180
black swan, 119
"black swan" event, 105
Black Swan, The (Taleb), 119, 120
bleeding disorder, 172
body mass index (BMI), 54
Bogen, Joseph, 242
books, stories or, 9–10
Boorstin, Daniel, 125
Boston University School of Medicine, 178
boundaries
   fluidity of, 174
   trespass, 174
bovine spongiform encephalopathy (BSE), 146–47
Box, George E. P., 114
Boxing, head injury, 253
Bragg, W. L., 108
brain
   expectations, 4
   toxic effects of metals on, 180
brain pathology, Parkinson's disease, 129
Brenner, Sydney, 134, 161, 211–13, 215, 226, 266, 267
   person to know, 162
Bretscher, M., 40
British Museum, London, 4
Broca, Paul, 204
Brodal, Alf, 226
Bronx Veterans Administration Medical Center, 112–13
Brookhaven National Labs, 217
Browning, Robert, 179
Brown-Sequard, Charles-Eduard, 225
Buddha, Gautama, 102, 180
Buddhism, 157
Buddhist proverb, 172–73
Budinger, Thomas, 185, 226
burnout, 191
Butler, Samuel, 255

Caenorhabditis elegans, 162
caffeine exposure, pregnancy, 119
calcification, 141
calcium homeostasis, 141
California Institute of Technology, 242
Cambridge Dictionary, 207
Cambridge University, 185
cancer, data collection, 225

cannibalism, 14, 243
Canon of Medicine, The (Avicenna), 187–88
carbon monoxide, patient visit, 31
cardiac arrhythmia, 99
Carlson, Arvid, 218
Case Against Reality, The (Hoffman), 3
Case of the Frozen Addicts, The (Langston), 245
Case Western Reserve University, 126
Cecil, Russell, 188
cell, term, 196
cerebral blood flow, 240
cerebrospinal fluid cytology, 241
Chain, Ernst Boris, 216, 217
Charcot, Jean Marie, 62
Charcot, Jean-Martin, 20, 145, 232
　person to know, 145
Charcot-Marie-Tooth disease, 62
Charnia masoni, 134
ChatGTP, 87
　artificial intelligence (AI) system, 183
Chinese proverb, 62
chorea, 62, 224–25
Christie, Agatha, 9
chronic traumatic encephalopathy (CTE), 253
Clark, David B., 123, 212
Clarke, Arthur C., 131
clinical experience, 74
　learning, 74
clinical significance, 169
clinicians, making contributions without a laboratory, 245–46
Coase, Ronald, 239
cognitive dysfunction, lead poisoning, 29–30
cognitive function, relevance in medicine, 78
cognitive processing, limits of capacity, 161
collaboration, research, 230
collaborative intelligence, 87
Columbia University, 197
Columbus, Christopher, 122
commission bias, 133
communication, patients, 92–93
compassion
　definition, 257
　inhibition by fear, 257
　intellectualization limiting, 26–28
　Judaism teaching, 258
　listening and being there, 258
　meditation, 258
　natural disaster, 258
　for ourselves, 257
　part of fundamental nature, 257–58
compassion fatigue, 191
competence, 78
confirmation bias, 132, 134
conscious ignorance, 53. *See also* ignorance
consent form, 78

Consilience (Wilson), 5
context
　care, 82–84
　definition, 84
　role in healthcare, 83
continental displacement, concept of, 212
continental drift, 212
Cooper, Irving, 245
Copernicus, 123
copying others, 133
Cornell University, 253
Coronel, Jason, 171
corticosteroids, 114
Cotzias, George, 208, 217, 218
　person to know, 218
Covey, Stephen, 31
COVID pandemic (2020–2022), 183
　unvaccinated people and, 256
cowpox, 216
crampons, 132
creeping paralysis, Parkinson's disease, 62
Creutzfeldt-Jakob disease, 63, 105, 214, 243
Crick, Francis, 162, 211–12, 224–25
　person to know, 227
Critchley, McDonald, 26
critical thinking
　asking questions and paying attention, 265
　observation for, 19–20
　paying attention, 55
　practicing, 267
　providing humane healthcare, 86–88
　thinking deeply, 99–102
CT scans, 173
cultural beliefs, older people, 261
Curie, Marie, 203
Curie, Pierre, 203
Cushing, Harvey, 196, 197
　person to know, 46
Cushing's syndrome, 45–46
cyanide, 41

Dalai Lama, 257
Dale, Sir Henry, 108
Dalton, Francis, 54, 237
Dandy, Walter, 197
Darwin, Charles, 104, 217
Darwin, Francis, 217
Darwin's theory of evolution, 134
data, information toxicity, 54–55
data sharing, availability of, 259
data torturing, 238
"Days" (Larkin), 157
day-tight compartments, 157
Debre, Patrice, 19–20
Debris, P., 183
deep brain stimulation, Parkinson's disease, 194

Deepwater Horizon, 127
defibrillator, cardiac resuscitation, 250
delirious ravings, 212
dementia, 194–95
   Alzheimer's disease, 63, 76
   cases of, 65
   forms of, 191
   patient with, 21–22
denial, illness or disability, 80–81
depression, 72, 266
dermatologist, 172
desirability bias, 133
diagnosis
   etiology, 46
   evaluation of patient, 45–46
   fundamental three-step approach, 45–46
   localization, 46
   momentum, 133
   signs and symptoms, 45
diagnostic testing, paying attention to assumptions, 240–42
diet, 190
Digoxin, 30–31
disability, denial of, 80–81
disease, evolutionary aspects of, 151–53
diversity, research, 230
Don't Think of an Elephant (Lakoff), 33, 36
Dopamine, Parkinson's disease, 217
Down syndrome, 24–25
   positron emission tomography (PET), 241
Drosophila (fruit flies), 146, 221
Dubos, Rene, 221–22
Duke University, 126

Easter Sunday, 107
Eccles, Sir John, 153
Edelman, Gerald, 4–5
Eder, Montague, 259
educator, responsibilities, 198–99
Ehrlich, Paul, 138, 178
   person to know, 138
Eijkman, Christiaan, 208–9
   person to know, 209
Einstein, Albert, 113, 122, 127, 147, 211
electroencephalogram (EEG), 56, 129, 228
electromyography (EMG), 16–17
Elizabeth I (Queen), 142
Emanuel, Ezekiel, 262–63
emergency room, 45
   facture of cervical spine, 65
   physical exams, 37–38
Emerson, Ralph Waldo, 177, 213, 269
emotional incontinence, 27–28
emotional intelligence, 144, 159
empathy, 144
empathy fatigue, 191

empirical, definition, 110
empirical evaluation, 116
encoding, 159
endocrine disease, 172
endocrine disturbances, 172
endocrinology, 225
end-of-life care, 22
Engel, G. L., 82
entorhinal, 241–42
environmental exposure, 152
epidemic, kuru, 243
epigenetics, 60
epilepsy, 214
   intractable, 241
episodic memory, 161–62
Epstein-Barr virus, 224–25
Erewhon (Butler), 255
errors
   medication, 94–95
   smart people making, 126–28
Escherichia coli, 146
Essay on the Shaky Palsy, The (Parkinson), 246
etiology, 90, 91
   diagnosis, 46
   mnemonic VITAMINS ABCD, 46, 47
   pathogenesis and, 47–48
Eucken, Rudolf, 111
euphemism(s), 35
   term, 35
evaluation, step in diagnosis, 45–46
evidence, intuition and, 110
evolution, 151, 266
   human, 3
evolutionary factors, 152
example, learning from a bad, 202
executive functions, 159
expectations, dependence on, 6–7
experience, patient's, 21–23
experimental bias, 235
experimenter bias, 141–42
experiments, research, 224–26
explicit denial, 80, 81

facts, theory and, 211–13
"false-negative" test, 34, 64
falsification principle, Popper proposing, 267
family history, interview including, 62
Faulkner, William, 195
Feinstein, Alvan, 230, 231
ferocity
   concept of, 14
   healthcare, 13–14
   pursuit of scientific objectives, 14
Ferry Catastrophe, 127
Feyerabend, Paul, 208, 211, 254
Feynman, Richard, 174, 213

fierce, 11
fishing expedition(s)
  investigations, 129
  scientific project as, 129
Fleming, Alexander, 194, 216
  person to know, 217
Florey, Sir Howard Walter, 216, 217
focus, 180–81
folk remedies, 95
Food and Drug Administration (FDA), 94
Fooled by Randomness (Talib), 133
Forest People, The (Turnbull), 7
form of denial, 131–32
Fox, Nicola, 11
framing, 33
  bias, 132
  medicine, 34
  regulations, 33–34
Frankl, Viktor, 66, 152, 163, 164
  person to know, 153
Freeman, Walter, 137–38
Freud, Sigmund, 163
friendly fire, term, 34–35
Fuller, Solomon Carter, 178
  person to know, 179
Fulton, John, 196
functional magnetic resonance imaging (fMRI), 240, 252–53

Gajdusek, Daniel Carleton, 14, 208, 243
  person to know, 244
Galen of Pergamon, 187–88
Galileo, 53, 82, 123, 127, 212
ganglion cysts, 226
Gardner, Howard, 144
Gawande, Atul, 14
Gazzaniga, Michael, 241
Gehry, Frank, 219–20
Geiger, H. Jack, 249, 250
  person to know, 250
genes, *Homo sapiens*, 3
genetics, 58–59
genetic testing, 49
genotype, 114–15
germ theory of disease, Pasteur and Lister, 82–83
Geula, Changiz, 222
God's will, 255
Goldman-Rakic, Patricia S., 203
gold standard, test, 35
Goleman, Daniel, 144
Gomez, Carlos, 40
gratefulness, 176
gratitude, 176
Grinker, Roy, 174
Groopman, Jerome, 18, 183, 257

group think, 253

Hachinski, Vladimir, 39
Hadlow, William, 243
Hallervorden, Julius, 252
Hallervorden-Spatz disease, 252
hallucination, 87–88
haloperidol, 41
Halsted, William, 196
  person to know, 197
hand-washing practices, mandatory, 82–83
happiness, 176
Harvard Medical School, 18, 25, 93
Harvard University, 13
Head, Harry, 225
head injury, boxing and American football, 253
health, paying attention to, 190–92
healthcare, challenges to ability to provide humane, 86–88
heart disease, oral health as risk factor, 66–67
heavy metals, toxic exposure, 60–61
Helicobacter pylori, 13–14, 124–25
  peptic ulcers, 193, 211, 217, 225
hemi-inattention, 21, 26
herbal products, 94
Herbert, Frank, 145
herbicides, toxic exposure, 60
herd mentality, 133
herpes zoster (shingles), 37–38, 66
Heschel, Abraham Joshua, 72, 86, 106
Hillary, Sir Edmund, 143
hindsight bias, 134–35
Hippocrates, 254
Hippocratic Oath, 233
histology, 223
HIV/AIDS pandemic, 105
HMS Camperdown, 126
Hoffman, Albert, 225
Hoffman, Donald, 3
Hofrath, Eduard, 84
Holmes, Oliver Wendell, Jr., 52
Holmes, Oliver Wendell, Sr., 120, 188
  person to know, 120
Holocaust, 153, 163, 252
homeostasis, 42
Homer, 255
Homo sapiens
  brain evolution in, 5
  genes, 3
Hooke, Robert, 196
Hopi Indians, languages, 33
Hopkins, Sir Frederick, 185
Hornykiewicz, Oleh, 217, 218
Horvitz, Robert, 212–13
How Doctors Think (Groopman), 18
Hubel, David, 242

human behavior, deserving their suffering, 255
human evolution, sensory abilities, 3
human genetics, 193
human health, denial of illness, 80
humility
    intellectual, 52
    See also ignorance
Hunter College, 112–13
Huntington's disease, 62
    etiology of, 47
Huxley, Aldous, 4, 8
hypertension, taking drugs for, 58
hyperthyroidism, 180
hypothyroidism, 180

ichthyology, 193
ideas
    assumptions, 149–50
    being first in, 216–17
    bias against new, 132
ignorance
    admitting to, 51–53
    being aware of your, 52
    conscious, 53
    intellectual humility, 52
    okay to be wrong, 122
illness, denial of, 80–81
Illness as Metaphor (Sontag), 255
illusion, language, 33
imaginary box, 112
imagination
    creativity, 147
    Einstein, 113
    not being afraid of your, 146–47
    thinking outside the box, 112
imaging procedures, disease detection, 50
immunization, cowpox and smallpox, 216
immunology, 138, 223
implicit bias, 137
implicit denial, 80, 81
incidentaloma/incidentalomas, 56, 228
"Indians," 122
infectious diseases, morbidity and mortality of, 260
inflammation, 149
information
    getting to know patient, 71–72
    investigations, 49–50
    not believing everything you read, 124–25
    recognizing intellectual ancestors, 196
    telling the truth, 76–77
    toxicity, 54–55, 259
in-group bias, 133
Institutional Review Board, 253
Insulin, discovery of, 225
Integrative Action of the Nervous System, The (Sherrington), 233

intellectual humility, 52
intellectualization, 26
    limiting compassion, 26–28
intelligence
    aspects of, 144
    being smart is not enough, 144
    concept of, 144
interest, getting to know patient, 71–72
interferons, 151
International Physicians for the Prevention of Nuclear War (IPPNW), 249
International Physiological Congress, 185
intervertebral disc disease, 105
interview, family history and, 62
intimidation, overcoming, of professionals in medicine and science, 185–86
Introduction to Experimental Medicine (Bernard), 42
intuition
    definition, 110
    value of, 110
Inuit peoples, languages, 33
investigation(s)
    information, 49–50
    on knowing the answer, 228–29
    productive fishing expeditions, 129
ischemia, 226

Jackson, Brian, 129
Jackson, John Hughlings, 171
    person to know, 171
Jacob, Francois, 139
James, William, 4, 6, 28, 57, 139, 158, 163, 171, 192, 242
    person to know, 8
Japan
    age discrimination, 262
    average age of population, 261
Jenner, Edward, 216
Johns Hopkins Hospital, 14, 197
Johnson, Samuel, 33
Jordan, Barry, 253
Journal of Clinical Investigation (journal), 112
Journal of Neurological Sciences (journal), 245
Journal of Neuro-Ophthalmology (journal), 199
Journal of Physiology (journal), 232
Journal of the American Medical Association (journal), 25, 76, 84
joy, 176
    compassion, 257
Joynt, Robert, 129
Judaism, teaching compassion, 258
judgment, 159

Kaiser Wilhelm Institute for Brain Research, 252
Kandel, Eric, 262–63

Kanehiro, Takaki, 208–9
Kant, Immanuel, 229
Kapitsa, Peter, 233
Kariko, Katalin, 183
karma, idea of, 255
Karolinska Institute, 124–25
Katz, Sir Bernard, 123, 237
Kekulé, August, 108
Kentucky Spinal Cord and Head Injury Research Board, 136–37
Klein, Autumn, 79
Koch, Robert, 138, 196, 209
  person to know, 139
Koch's postulates, 139
Koestler, Arthur, 207
Kohler, Wolfgang, 174
Kornfield, Jack, 190, 219
Kraepelin, Emil, 178, 194
  person to know, 194–95
Kreutzfeldt-Jakob disease, 208
Kubla Khan (Coleridge), 107
Kuhn, Thomas, 207–8
kuru, 146, 208, 243
  transmissibility of, 14

Laennec, Rene, 132
Lakoff, George, 33, 36
  person to know, 36
laminectomy, 114
Lamm, Richard, 262
Lancet (journal), 252
Langer, Robert, 18
Langston, William, 13–14, 245
  Parkinson's disease, 119
language, 33, 159
Larkin, Philip, 157
Lashley, Karl, 241
L-dihydroxyphenylalanine (L-dopa), precursor of dopamine, 218
lead poisoning, patient visit, 29–30
learning
  accepting help of others, 187–88
  clinical experience, 74
  critical reading of literature, 168–69
  educator responsibilities, 198–99
  enhancing capacity for, 159–61
  focus but not too much, 180–81
  history of medicine and science, 193–94
  learning from bad example, 202
  not being intimidated by professionals, 185–86
  from patients, 24–25
  paying attention to health and stress, 190–92
  persistence and tenacity, 182–83
  public speaking, 200–1
  pursuit of, 11
  recognizing intellectual ancestors, 196
  salesperson, 200–1
  variability in styles of, 159–61
Lessell, Simmons, 199
Letters to a Young Scientist (Wilson), 172, 219
leucotomy, 138
levodopa, Parkinson's disease, 208
Levy, Barry, 249–50
Lewy, Frederick, 129, 178
  person to know, 130
Lewy body dementia, 130
Lewy body disease, 178
listening
  art of, to patients, 16–18
  communication, 92
  compassion, 258
  patient visit, 29–31
Listening for What Matters (Weiner and Schwarz), 84
Lister, Joseph, 84, 149, 197, 207
  germ theory of disease, 83
literature, critical reading of, 168–69
"liver enzymes," 35
localization, diagnosis, 46
Loewi, Otto, 107
  person to know, 108
logic, definition, 107
logical fallacy, 222
logotherapy school of psychoanalysis, 153
London Times (newspaper), 132
lost actors, bias of, 143
Lost Art of Healing, The (Lown), 100–1
Lost in the 20th Century (Szent-Györgyi), 223
Lown, Bernard, 59, 72, 100–1, 249, 250
  person to know, 250
Lown Institute, 59
lymph nodes, 226
lysergic acid diethylamide (LSD), 225

McCulloch, Warren, 241
McHugh, Thomas, 217
Macleod, John, 233
magnetic resonance imaging (MRI), 56, 87
Maimonides, Moses, 23
Mallory, George, 228
Man's Search for Meaning (Frankl), 153, 163
Marie, Pierre, 62
Mars, NASA mission, 126
Marshall, Barry, 13–14, 124–25, 193, 217, 225
Mason, Roger, 134
Mathematics, science and medicine, 219
Maxwell, James Clerk, 53
Mechnikoff, Elie, 137
  person to know, 138
Medawar, Peter, 224–25
medical school, not believing everything you read, 124–25

medications
    being attentive to, 94–95
    compliance with, 41
    patient visit, 30–31
medicine
    cognitive function, 78
    intelligence of researchers, 219–20
    learning from history of, 193–94
    neurologists, 170–71
    not being intimidated by professionals, 185–86
    profession of, 176
    science and, 160
    tendency for healthcare workers to blame patients, 255
meditation, 190
    practice of, 257
memory, 4–5, 159, 169
    competence, 78
    stress in, 266
memory disorders clinic, 22–23
meningococcal meningitis, 37
Menninger, Karl, 39, 255
mental hygiene, term, 137–38
mental status exam, 37
metaphor, figure of speech, 35–36
Metchnikoff, Elie, 138
Meyer, Adolph, 137–38
microbiology, 58–59, 174
microsurgery, development of, 102
"milieu interieur," term, 42
Mills, J. L., 238
mineralization, 141
mistakes, smart people making, 126–28
models
    animal, 114
    mouse, 114–15
Moniz, António Egas, 138
Montefiore Medical Center, 249–50
Moskva, Russian Navy, 35
motion sickness, 151
motor neuron disease (MND), 145
    Alzheimer's disease and, 60–61
Mount Sinai Hospital, 41, 144
Mount Sinai School of Medicine, 196, 245
mouse, visual system in thalamus, 222–23
mouse models, 114–15
    Alzheimer's disease, 115
MPTP (1-methyl-4-phenyl-1,2,3,6-tetrahydropyridine), 61
MRI. *See* magnetic resonance imaging (MRI)
multiple reserves, 66
multiple sclerosis (MS), 133
    risk of, 101
multitasking, 160
Musil, Robert, 269
My Life in Science (Brenner), 161

myocardial infarction, 37
myth of progress, 259–60

Nagel, Thomas, 3
NASA mission, Mars, 126
National Institute of Aging (NIA), 141, 214
National Institute of Mouse Biology (NIMB), 221
National Institute of Neurological Disorders and Stroke (NINDS), 214
National Institutes of Health (NIH), 214, 221, 243, 244, 252–53
National Library of Medicine, 229, 265
naturalist, 180
Nature (journal), 124, 168, 229, 244
nausea, 151
Nazi Party, 252
Nazism, 130
Negus, Tina, 134
Nesse, Randolph, 152, 153
Neuroimage (journal), 235
neuroimaging, 223
neurologists, 170–71
    definition, 170
neurology, 78, 173, 174
    psychiatry and, 214
Neurology (journal), 144
neuromyelitis optica (NMO), 265
neuronal degeneration, nootropics and, 101
neuropsychiatry, 178
neurosurgery, 78
neurotoxin MPTP (1-methyl-4-phenyl-1,2,3,6-tetrahydropyridine), 245
Neurotree figure, 196
New England Journal of Medicine (journal), 16–17, 64, 250, 256
Newton, Isaac, 105–6, 196
New York Madison Square Garden, 253
New York State Athletic Commission, 253
New York Times (newspaper), 131
New York University, 168, 245
Nietzsche, Friedrich, 36
Nin, Anaïs, 8
Nissl, Franz, 178
nitrous oxide, 149
nocebo effect, 75, 94–95
noncompliance, 58
nootropics, Alzheimer's disease and, 101
Northwestern University, 222
nosology, 194

Oberlin College, 242
observation
    critical thinking, 19–20
    expectations, 4
    preparing for unexpected, 41–42
observations, learning, 170

observer, suggestions for being a good, 19
Occam's razor, 105–6, 123
older people, ageism and, 261–63
olfactory detection, Alzheimer's disease, 241–42
OpenAI, 87
Oppenheim, Herman, 178
optimism bias, 135
oral health, as risk factor, 66–67
organotherapy, 225
organs, functions of, 170
Origin of Continents and Oceans, The (Wegener), 212
Osler, William, 16, 38, 59, 61, 72, 95, 157, 161, 173, 188
   person to know, 14
   "The Student Life," 11–12
Ottoman Empire, 216
"out of the box" thinking, 112
overconfidence bias, 132
overspecialization, 172
Oxford English Dictionary, 207, 240, 257
Oxford English Dictionary Online, 131
Oxford University, 194

pain fibers, 170
paleontology, 193, 246
pantothenate kinase-associated neurodegeneration, 252
paradigms, filtering perception, 213
paradigm shift, term, 207–8, 209
parenteral, term, 203–4
Parkinson, James, 232, 246
   person to know, 246
Parkinson's disease, 13–14, 25, 105, 146
   acute onset of, 245
   "creeping paralysis," 62
   data collection, 225
   deep brain stimulation, 194
   dihydroxyphenylalaine (DOPA), 217
   high doses of L-dopa, 218
   investigations on, 129
   Langston, 119
   levodopa, 208
   localization of pathology in, 130
   past beliefs on, 124
   pathogenesis of, 47
   treatment, 225
passion, search for, and follow it, 165–66
passionate disinterest, 133
passive reading, 168
Pasteur, Louis, 19–20, 42, 127, 138, 139, 183, 230
   germ theory of disease, 15, 82–83
   person to know, 183
   tenacity, 182
pathogenesis, etiology and, 47–48
pathology, 58–59

pathophysiology, 90
patient(s)
   attentive to, and knowledgeable, 58–59
   cognitive function, 78
   communication with, 92–93
   compassion for, 257
   denial of illness or disability, 80–81
   distinctiveness of, 104
   educator responsibilities, 198
   experience of, 21–23
   fierce in working for benefit of, 11, 12–13
   getting to know as person, 71–72
   health of, 41
   interactions, 7–8
   key elements of visit, 29–31
   learning from, 24–25
   learning from clinical experience, 74
   listening to, 16–18
   placebo response, 75
   preparing for unexpected, 41–42
   responsibility for caring for, 79
   telling the truth whenever possible, 76–77
   tendency of healthcare workers to blame, 255
   three-step approach to diagnosis, 45–46
   treating, 56
Peabody, Francis, 93
   person to know, 93
pedestrians, expectations, 4
Peebles, James, 108
penicillin
   discovery of, 217
   Fleming, 194, 216
Penicillium, Fleming, 216
peptic ulcer, 124–25
   Helicobacter pylori, 217
peptic ulcer disease, *Helicobacter pylori*, 193, 225
perception(s)
   dependence on expectations, 6–7
   role of experience in, 7
   sensory systems, 3
   world, 4
periodontitis, 100
Perry, John, 161
persistence, tenacity and, 182–83
Perutz, Max, 42
pesticides, toxic exposure, 60
Pfizer, 122–23
phagocytosis, 137
pharmacodynamics, 58
pharmacokinetics, 58
pharmacology, 58–59
phenotype, 114–15
phenylketonuria (PKU), pathophysiology of, 90
physical exam, 37–38
physical exercise, stress, 191
physical therapy, 72

physical touch, importance of, 39
physician, caring for patient, 79
Physicians for Social Responsibility (PSR), 249
physiology, 214
pigmentary retinal degeneration, 24
placebo effect(s), 75, 94–95, 235–36
plasticity, 72
Plato, 107
pluripotent, 167
pneumonia, symptoms and signs of, 64
Poincare, Henri, 107, 269
Popper, Karl, 267
positron emission tomography (PET), 49, 87, 173, 201, 226
  Alzheimer's disease, 185
  Down syndrome, 241
Post-It Sticky Notes, 122
posttraumatic stress disorder (PTSD), 55, 191
  questions about, 266
Prager, Katrin, 223
pregnancy
  alcohol intake during, 118
  caffeine exposure, 119
presenile, 194–95
presenile dementia, 194
Principles and Practice of Medicine, The (Osler), 14, 188
prion, term, 216–17
pro choice, 33–34
progress, myth of, 259–60
progressive dementia, 173
pro-life, framing, 33–34
prostate cancer, choice of therapies, 78
Prusiner, Stanley, 14, 216–17
pseudobulbar palsy, 27–28
psychiatric diagnoses, 83
psychiatry, 78, 174
  neurology and, 214
psychology, 78
psychotherapy, 91
public speaking, stress of, 201
publishing, educator responsibilities, 199
PubMed database, 149
puerperal fever, 82–83

questions
  asking professionals, 185–86
  asking with ferocity, 266
  critical thinking, 265
  formation of, 266
  learning, 160
quotations, nature of scientific endeavor, 269

Rabi, Isidore, 266
rabies, 31
racial bias, 137

radioimmunoassay, 112–13
radiology, 174
Ramon y Cajal, Santiago, 195, 220
rare events
  definition, 104
  occurrence(s), 63, 104–6
rational, 207
razor, term, 105–6
Reagan, Ronald, 80
recreational activities, patient visit, 29
regulations, word, 33–34
reification, 172–73
relaxation, 161
Remen, Naomi, 192
rendering, 146
Republic of Korea, average age of population, 261
research
  attention to assumptions for evaluations, 240–42
  attention to study design, data analysis, and statistics, 235–37
  being first in, 216–17
  bias, 141
  clinicians making contributions without a laboratory, 245–46
  diversity and collaboration, 230
  diversity of approaches, 221–23
  experimenting, 224–26
  importance of, 230
  importance of knowing the answers, 228–29
  researchers not needing to be brilliant, 219–20
  volunteers, 255
resilience, 66
resources, pursuing best, 178
responsibility, actions, 252–53
retrieval, 159
reverence for life, Schweitzer, 111
reverse causation, 238–39
right parietal lobe damage, 26–27
risk factors, 100
road rash, term, 34
rofecoxib, clinical trials, 259
Rosenhan, D. L., 83
Roy, Charles S., 193, 232
Royal Psychiatric Hospital, 178
rule out, phrase, 34
Rutherford, Lord Ernest, 237

Sacks, Oliver, 226
Sagan, Carl, 187
Salmonella, 31
salutogenesis, concept of, 66
sampling bias, 135
Santillan, Jessica, 126
Sapir, Edward, 33
Schilder, Paul, 203
Schopenhauer, Arthur, 111

Schwab, Robert, 25
Schwartz, Martin A., 52, 133, 269
Schwarz, A., 84
Schweitzer, Albert, 111, 166, 202
　person to know, 111
　"reverence for life," 111
science
　definition, 207
　disciplines of, 172
　diversity of approaches, 221–23
　intelligence of researchers, 219–20
　learning from history of, 193–94
　not being intimidated by professionals, 185–86
　study of everything, 214–15
Science (journal), 83, 87, 112, 168, 216–17
scientific endeavor, quotations on nature of, 269
scientific literature, not believing everything you read, 124–25
scientific paper, critical reading of, 168–69
Scientific Reports, 229
Scientific Revolution, 142
Scotland, Beethaeven, 253
scrapie, 146, 243
Scripps national spelling bee, 236
selective breeding, 165
self-serving bias, 133
semantic memory, 161–62
Semmelweis, Ignaz, 82–83, 120, 127, 149
　person to know, 84
senile dementia, 100
senile psychosis, 100
senility, 100, 261
sensory systems, 3
severe acute respiratory syndrome coronavirus 2 (SARS–CoV-2), 183
sexual history, patient visit, 30
shadowing, 11
Shaw, George Bernard, 176, 269
Sherrington, Sir Charles S., 193, 196, 232
　person to know, 233
shingles, herpes zoster, 66
Sidel, Victor, 249, 250
　person to know, 249–50
signs and symptoms, step in diagnosis, 45
sildenafil, 122–23
silence, 39
Silver, Spencer, 122
Simon, Herbert, 55
Sippy Diet, 52
Slovic, Paul, 258
smallpox, 216
"smart people make mistakes," principle of, 127–28
Smith, Huston, 258
social exposome, 83
social history, patient visit, 29

social medicine, concept of, 250
Society for Nuclear Medicine, 201
Socrates, 107
Solanaceae family of plants, 131
solvents, toxic exposure, 60, 61
somatic and psychic
　interrelations, 174
Sontag, Susan, 255
SpaceX Corporation, 35
spatial reasoning, 159
Spatz, Hugo, 252
specialization, pursuing, 165–66
specificity, 116–17
speech therapy, 72
Sperry, Roger W., 241
　person to know, 242
Spielmeyer, Walther, 178
spinal cord injury, 114
splinter hemorrhages, 64–65
Spurious Correlations, 236
Stanford University, 83, 161
Staphylococci, 217
Staphylococcus aureus, 216
Starship rocket, 35
statistical significance, 169
statistics, 238–39
status epilepticus, 38
Steck, Ueli, 132
Stetson, R. H., 242
Stevenson, Robert Louis, 107
Stockholm Harbor, 127
storage, memory, 159
stories, books or, 9–10
"stork legs," atrophy, 62
stress
　burnout, 191
　paying attention to, 190–92
　psychological, 191
stroke, 26, 153, 226
　drawing of tree by man with, 27f
　neurologist on causes, 99–100
　oral health as risk factor, 66–67
　right middle cerebral artery, 26
Structure of Scientific Revolutions, The (Kuhn), 207–8
"Student Life, The" (Osler), 11–12
students, ferocity in learning, 11
Sulston, John, 212–13
Sun, T., 168
sundowning, 76
supplements, patient visit, 30–31
survival, sensory abilities, 3
survivorship bias, 143
symptoms and signs, important significance of, 64–65
synapse, term, 233

Szent-Györgyi, Albert, 115, 180–81, 185, 221, 269
    person to know, 223

tabes dorsalis (syphilis), 225
Tagore, Rabindranath, 107, 123, 173, 176
Taleb, Nassim, 119, 120, 133
Taylor, Jill Bolte, 226
teaching, educator responsibilities, 198–99
temporal arteritis, 51
Temporarily Able-Bodied "TABs," 256
tenacious, word, 14
tenacity, persistence and, 182–83
Textbook (Kraepelin), 194
textbooks, 58
"theater" of war, 34–35
theories, facts and, 211–13
Thich Nhat Hanh, 190, 258
thinking
    concepts of outside the box, 112
    deeply, 99–102
    experimenting in research, 224–26
    freedom in, 112
    "out of the box," 112
    words influence thought, 33–35
Thoreau, Henry David, 165, 178, 179
thought. *See* thinking
3M Company, Minnesota, 122
Tononi, Giulio, 4–5
tonsils, 226
Tooth, Howard, 62
touch, importance of physical, 39
toxic exposures, 60–61, 255–56
toxicity, information, 54–55
treatment, patient visit, 30–31
Treg cells, 190
trespassing, 174
trichinosis, 48
Tryon, George, 126
tuberculosis, 139, 225
Tukey, John, 235, 237
Tulving, Endel, 159
    person to know, 161–62
Turkey-Syria earthquake (2023), natural disaster, 258
Turnbull, Colin, 7

Ukrainian missiles, 35
ulnar nerve, 170
Unaging (Friedland), 66
unilateral neglect, 21, 26
    drawing of tree by man with stroke, 27f
unilateral neurological deficit, 21
University of California, Berkeley, 208, 226
University of California, Davis, 185
University of Chicago, 242
University of Hawaii, 268

University of Illinois, 112–13
University of Oregon, 258
University of Pittsburgh, 79
University of Rochester, 129
University of Toronto, 233
Urey, Harold, 209
US Alzheimer's Association, 116
US Army, helmets and facial wounds, 101
US Centers of Disease Control, 118
US Department of Agriculture, 147
US Department of Health, 261
US Food and Drug Administration (FDA), 116
US National Academies of Science, Engineering and Medicine, 118
US National Library of Medicine, 112–13, 115
US Supreme Court, 120

vaccinations, 182
vaccines, mRNA for COVID pandemic, 183
Varmus, Harold, 196
Vasa (warship), 127
vestibular system, vision and, 151
Veterans Administration hospital, 16–17, 133, 135
Vibrios, Pasteur, 19–20
Victor, Maurice, 13
Victoria (flagship), 126
video-game palsy, 16–17
Vietnam War, 250
Virchow, Rudolf, 14, 82–83, 127, 128, 196
    person to know, 15
viruses, vaccines against, 182
vision, vestibular system and, 151
visit, elements of patient, 29–31
vitamins
    attentive to, 94
    discover of vitamin C, 185
    patient visit, 30–31
    sun exposure and vitamin D, 101
VITAMINS ABCD, 46
    etiology and pathogenesis, 47–48
    mnemonic for etiologies, 47
    use of, 48
von Behring, Emil, 137, 138, 139
    person to know, 138
von Braun, Werhner, 209
von Monakow, Constantin, 178
von Neumann, John, 211

Walter Reed Army Medical Service Graduate School, 244
Warren, Robin, 13–14, 124–25, 217
water, ancestor searching for, 4
Watson, James, 162, 211–12, 227
Wegener, Alfred, 178, 212
Weiner, S. J., 84
Weissman, Drew, 183

Wells, Horace, 149
Wernicke, Carl, 203–4
   person to know, 204
Wernicke's aphasia, 204
Wernicke's encephalopathy, 203–4
What Mad Pursuit (Crick), 227
Where My Caravan Has Rested (Kaplan), 179
White supremacy, 137
white swan event, 120
Whorf, Benjamin, 33
Wiesel, Torsten, 242
Wilkins, Maurice, 227
William of Ockham, 105–6
Wilson, Edward O., 5, 166, 172, 219, 220
   person to know, 5
Wolberg, Lewis, 39

Woodcock, Janet, 116
words, influencing thought, 33–35
workplace, toxic exposure, 60
world, perceptions of, 4
writing, educator responsibilities, 199

Yalow, Rosalyn, 112, 113
   person to know, 112–13
Yamanaka, Shinya, 166
   person to know, 167
Yanagimachi, Ryuzo, 267
   person to know, 268
Yersinia pestis, 31
Yoshikawa, Toshikazu, 10

Zinsser, William, 199